MEDICAL SETTING CONSIDERATIONS
for the
SPEECH-LANGUAGE PATHOLOGIST

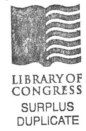

Medical Speech-Language Pathology
Series Editors
Kristie A. Spencer, PhD, CCC-SLP
Jacqueline Daniels, MA, CCC-SLP, CBIS

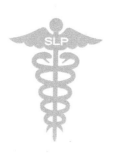

MEDICAL SETTING
CONSIDERATIONS
for the
SPEECH-LANGUAGE
PATHOLOGIST

Kristie A. Spencer, PhD, CCC-SLP
Jacqueline Daniels, MA, CCC-SLP, CBIS

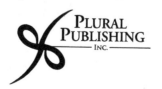

PLURAL
PUBLISHING
INC.

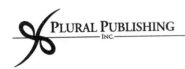

5521 Ruffin Road
San Diego, CA 92123

e-mail: information@pluralpublishing.com
Website: http://www.pluralpublishing.com

Typeset in 11/13 Adobe Garamond by Flanagan's Publishing Services, Inc.
Printed in the United States of America by Integrated Books International

For permission to use material from this text, contact us by
Telephone: (866) 758-7251
Fax: (888) 758-7255
e-mail: permissions@pluralpublishing.com

Every attempt has been made to contact the copyright holders for material originally printed in another source. If any have been inadvertently overlooked, the publishers will gladly make the necessary arrangements at the first opportunity.

Library of Congress Cataloging-in-Publication Data

Names: Spencer, Kristie A., editor. | Daniels, Jacqueline, editor.
Title: Medical setting considerations for the speech-language pathologist /
    [edited by] Kristie A. Spencer, Jacqueline Daniels.
Other titles: Medical speech-language pathology (Series)
Description: San Diego, CA : Plural Publishing, [2020] | Series: Medical
    speech-language pathology | Includes bibliographical references and index.
Identifiers: LCCN 2019002630| ISBN 9781635501032 (alk. paper) | ISBN
    1635501032 (alk. paper)
Subjects: | MESH: Language Disorders | Speech-Language Pathology
Classification: LCC RC423 | NLM WL 340.2 | DDC 616.85/5—dc23
LC record available at https://lccn.loc.gov/2019002630

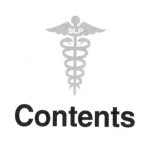

Contents

Series Overview

The Medical Speech-Language Pathology book series provides graduate students, clinicians, and clinical researchers with functional, comprehensive material to enhance practice in a medical setting. The books are designed to bolster transdisciplinary knowledge through infusion of information from neurology, pharmacology, radiology, otolaryngology, and other related disciplines. They capture our current understanding of complex clinical populations, often encountered in medical settings, and offer information to guide evaluation and management strategies. For each clinical population, case studies are used to promote application and integration of the material. Moreover, the handbooks are richly supplemented with figures, tables, and patient samples to enhance accessibility of the information. Each book in the series is authored by experienced professionals and content experts who are able to transform the research literature into clinically applicable and digestible information. The authors integrate theory and practice in a succinct manner, allowing immediate application to everyday practice. This book series advances the medical speech-language pathology community by merging fundamental concepts, clinical strategies, and current theories with research evidence, with the goal of fostering outstanding clinical practice and clinical research.

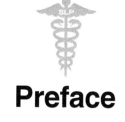

Preface

The overarching goal of this book is to foster an appreciation of the unique skill set and knowledge base needed by a medical speech-language pathologist (SLP). The chapters contain information applicable to a broad range of medical and rehabilitation settings, while delving deeper into complex topics that merit extra attention, such as neuroimaging methods and medication side effects. Readers will come to appreciate the many roles and responsibilities of the speech-language pathologist in the medical setting, across the continuum of care. They will gain familiarity with broader organizational issues, such as accreditation, billing, and medical team members, as well as the specific clinical populations often encountered in medical settings, such as individuals with Parkinson's disease, delirium, or tongue cancer. Throughout the book, case studies are used to highlight the role of the medical SLP, and to underscore the remarkably dynamic and complex caseloads encountered by the medical SLP.

Contributors

Matina Balou, PhD, CCC-SLP, BCS-S
Assistant Professor
Department of Otolaryngology–Head and
Neck Surgery
NYU School of Medicine
NYU Langone Health
New York City, New York
Chapter 2

Alexandra E. Brandimore, PhD, CCC-SLP
Assistant Professor
Communication Sciences and Disorders
University of South Florida
Tampa, Florida
Chapter 4

Jacqueline Daniels, MA, CCC-SLP, CBIS
Lecturer, Speech-Language Pathology
Certified Brain Injury Specialist
Department of Speech and Hearing Sciences
University of Washington
Seattle, Washington
Chapter 5

Angela M. Hill, PharmD, CRPh
Professor and Chair
Department of Pharmacotherapeutics and
Clinical Research
Associate Dean of Clinical Practice
University of South Florida College of
Pharmacy
Tampa, Florida
Chapter 4

Doreen Kelly Izaguirre, MA, CCC-SLP
Speech-Language Pathology Clinical
Education Manager, Rush University
Faculty, Rush University, Department of
Communication Disorders and Sciences

Speech-Language Pathologist, Rush
University Medical Center
Chicago, Illinois
Chapter 2

Rene Ruzicka Kanadet, MS, CCC-SLP
Speech Pathologist
Edward Hines Jr. VA Hospital
Hines, Illinois
Clinical Development Leader, Speech
Pathology
KatieBug Therapy, Ltd
Naperville, Illinois
Chapter 2

Jacqueline Laures-Gore, PhD, CCC-SLP
Associate Professor
Department of Communication Sciences
and Disorders
Georgia State University
Atlanta, Georgia
Chapter 1

Linda I. Shuster, PhD, CCC-SLP
Professor
Department of Speech, Language, and
Hearing Sciences
Western Michigan University
Kalamazoo, Michigan
Chapter 3

Kristie A. Spencer, PhD, CCC-SLP
Professor
Associate Chair, Graduate Program
Coordinator
Department of Speech and Hearing Sciences
University of Washington
Seattle, Washington
Chapters 2 and 5

Katlynd Marie Sunjic, PharmD
Assistant Professor
Department of Pharmacotherapeutics and
    Clinical Research
University of South Florida College of
    Pharmacy
Tampa, Florida
Chapter 4

Sheeba Varghese Gupta, MPharm, PhD
Assistant Professor
University of South Florida College of
    Pharmacy
Tampa, Florida
Chapter 4

Acknowledgments

We would like to acknowledge our many mentors and students across the years who have shaped us into the professionals we are today. A heartfelt thank you to our families for their patience and understanding while we spent many evenings and weekends on the book. And a very special thanks to Kalie Koscielak, the Associate Acquisitions Editor, for her endless patience and guidance.

This book is dedicated to the many individuals with medical and neurological challenges that we have met along our speech-language pathology journey. Thank you for helping us grow as clinicians, instructors, and researchers. We are forever inspired by your strength.

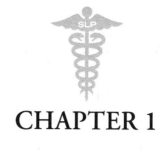

CHAPTER 1

The Medical Environment: Team Members and Organizational Issues

Jacqueline Laures-Gore

INTRODUCTION

Medical speech-language pathologists work in a complex, constantly evolving health care system. Recent federal government changes to health care reform (Patient Protection and Affordable Care Act [PPACA], 2010) as well as earlier changes in the 1990s (e.g., Balanced Budget Act of 1997) within the United States have resulted in a medical care landscape that necessitates flexibility by the speech-language pathologist. Because debates about the funding of health care continue to exist in federal and state governments in the United States, it is most likely that changes to the health care system will persist. It is important for speech-language pathologists to understand this dynamic health care environment and become aware of the factors influencing service delivery to ensure speech-language services for individuals who need it. For example, only 55% of children who need voice, speech, language, or swallowing intervention services receive these services (National Institute on Deafness and Other Communication Disorders [NIDCD], 2016). Improving speech-language pathologist's knowledge about the complicated and dynamic health care environment will help the profession advocate for those individuals who need our services.

Speech-language pathologists are essential team members in diverse medical environments, and the recognition of their importance is increasing, as the profession's scope of practice becomes better understood by their colleagues. The title "speech-language pathology" captures the underlying medical basis of the profession as pathology indicates an organically based problem. However, speech and language impairments represent only a portion of the myriad challenges addressed by our profession. Speech-language pathologists also contribute to areas such as cognition, swallowing, voice, feeding, and aural rehabilitation. Indeed, this is a profession deeply rooted in medicine that is a crucial contributor to the successful outcomes of patients treated within the United States' health care system. However, the success of the profession and the patients they serve relies upon the other members of the medical environment. Speech-language pathologists support and interact with many other health care professionals in an interprofessional, collaborative manner.

This chapter outlines the roles and responsibilities of speech-language pathologists in the medical setting, describes the different health care environments in which they are employed, provides descriptions of other health care professionals with whom speech-language pathologists interact, and discusses the health care organization's structure and process, including billing procedures. Figure 1–1 provides a summary of the different facets of the speech-language pathologist in the medical setting as they are described below.

ROLES AND RESPONSIBILITIES OF THE SPEECH-LANGUAGE PATHOLOGIST

Across medical settings, the roles and responsibilities of speech-language pathologists are guided by the current American Speech-Language-Hearing Association (ASHA) Scope of Practice (ASHA, 2016). Practice areas describing service delivery of speech-language pathologists are contextualized within eight domains: (1) collaboration, (2) counseling, (3) prevention and wellness, (4) screening, (5) assessment, (6) treatment, (7) modalities, technology, and instrumentation, and (8) population and systems (e.g., improving

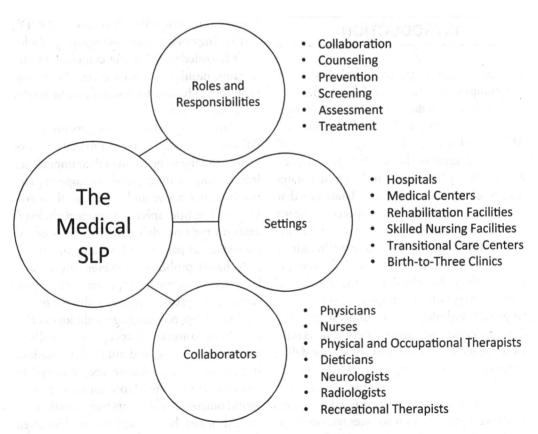

Figure 1–1. The many facets of the speech-language pathologist.

overall health of different clinical populations, improving the individual experience of those served, and decreasing the cost of services (ASHA, 2016). Although the service delivery domains are varied, they all relate to the speech-language pathologist's responsibility to consumers to improve their communication and swallowing skills. Moreover, all of these areas are situated within the International Classification of Functioning, Disability, and Health (ICF; World Health Organization, 2001), which provides a classification framework shared across disciplines, thus enabling better communication between health care professionals.

Speech-language pathologists work with a wide range of ages across an array of etiologies. For instance, these clinicians may assess and treat swallowing disorders in neonatal units or work with the palliative care needs experienced during the end of life associated with degenerative neurological diseases. Critically ill patients seen in the Intensive Care Unit (ICU) can be seen by speech-language pathologists for swallowing to determine safety, as well as to educate patient/family/staff. As the patient progresses through the continuum of care, including step-down units, rehabilitation centers, and long-term care facilities, the speech-language pathologist will continue to assess, treat, and educate. Although the medical environment changes, the role of the speech-language pathologist remains the same.

The continuum of care within the acute care setting includes the ICU where patients receive intense medical care targeting health stabilization. Within this setting, speech-language pathologists will be the first to assess swallowing function, cognitive, speech or language skills, and perhaps, become involved with tracheostomies and ventilators. The patient may then advance to a step-down unit, alternatively referred to as a progressive or intermediate care unit (American Association of Critical-Care Nurses, 2009; Stacy, 2011).

This concept was first introduced in the 1960s and is designed for hospitalized patients who do not need intensive medical care, but are not ready for the level of care in a typical hospital unit. Indeed, it is an intermediate stage of care defined by the nurse-to-patient ratio and the provision of organ support (Prin & Wunsch, 2014). With the improved medical stability of the patient at this stage, speech-language pathologists may be able to provide longer therapy sessions, addressing communication and/or swallowing issues identified during the ICU stay. Additionally, more in-depth patient and family education may occur. Following the step-down unit, patients may then advance to another unit in the hospital providing a lower nurse-to-patient ratio. After hospitalization, patients may be discharged to the home where they are prescribed outpatient or home health care services. The determination of these services is based on the patient's status as either homebound or able to get to an outpatient clinic for services. In the home environment, speech-language pathologists will continue to conduct dynamic assessment and address the established, and perhaps emerging, communication or swallowing impairments identified in the hospital setting. It may be determined that a person needs inpatient rehabilitation prior to release to home and, subsequently, the patient may stay in a rehabilitation center for intense daily multidisciplinary therapy. Within this environment, the speech-language pathologist will often be cotreating with other therapists to improve the outcomes of intervention. Alternatively, a patient may require a skilled nursing facility for transitional care while short-term rehabilitation services are provided, followed by either a return to home or more long-term care in a residential facility.

To address the complexity of the varied roles, responsibilities, patient populations, and medical settings, many speech-language pathologists seek additional certification beyond the Certificate of Clinical Competence (CCC) to demonstrate their training and expertise. Through the Clinical Specialty Certification program, overseen by the Clinical Certification in Audiology and Speech-Language Pathology, there are three specialty certificates offered, including (1) child language and language disorders; (2) fluency and fluency disorders; and (3) swallowing and swallowing disorders. There are specific requirements that speech-language pathologists must meet in order to be awarded the specialty certification (see http://www.asha.org/certification/specialty/). The Academy of Neurological Communication Disorders and Sciences provides Board Certification for speech-language pathologists specializing in neurologic communication disorders (see http://www.ancds.org/board-certification-process). Additionally, one may become a Certified Brain Injury Specialist through the Brain Injury Association of America. Speech-language pathologists may also pursue specialty training in techniques such as the Lee Silverman Voice Treatment (LSVT), Fiberoptic Endoscopic Evaluation of Swallowing (FEES), and Myofascial Release and Manual Therapy. Speech-language pathologists may seek out other specialty training depending upon the needs of their patients, environments, and the other members of the medical team.

THE MEDICAL TEAM

The collaboration between speech-language pathologists and other health care professionals is essential in the successful care of patients across medical settings. Speech-language pathologists consistently interact with physicians from different specialty and subspecialty areas, with nurses with a variety of education and certification levels, as well as dieticians, social workers, and mental health professionals, including psychologists and neuropsychologists. Although historically there has been the perception of a hierarchy between physicians, nurses, and allied health professionals, there is a cultural shift toward interdisciplinary or transdisciplinary patient-centered care that emphasizes collaboration and fostering of continuity of care (Freidson, 1970; Robinson, Callister, Bearing, & Dearing, 2008).

Important to a collaborative culture is the involvement of the speech-language pathologist in clinical rounds, team conferences, and care conferences. Clinical rounds are an opportunity for all members of the medical team to meet and discuss the issues faced by a given patient. One of the team members may present an overview of the patient's condition and current status, followed by other team members adding their perspective through the lens of their specialty. Family members and the patient may be in attendance. Similarly, during team or care conferences, the medical team meets to discuss the care of a patient; during these meetings, the family member and patient are encouraged to attend. These conferences include long-term plans for the care of the patient, thus involvement of the family is key. Typical members of the care team are outlined below.

Physicians

The speech-language pathologist works closely with physicians from a variety of specialty areas. The training of physicians includes four years of medical school, followed by a residency ranging from three to seven years, potentially followed by a fellowship, and then certification or licensure (Association of American Medical Colleges [AAMC], 2018). A 2015 survey conducted by the AAMC indicates that there are over 40 physician specialties in the United States health care system (AAMC, 2016). Table 1–1 provides a listing of common physician specialties. One such specialty is hospitalists. Hospitalists are physicians who stay within the hospital to provide inpatient medicine for patients. The inception of this specialty was in response to the emergence of managed care and changes to Medicare (Wachter & Goldman, 1996, 2016). This model has led to decreased hospital costs and length of stay in hospitals. With an increasing trend of their use since the mid-1990s, there are now an estimated 50,000 hospitalists in the United States (Landrigan, Conway, Edwards, & Srivastava, 2006; Rachoin et al., 2012; Wachter & Goldman, 2016). Hospitalists have been a mainstay in other health care systems, such as Canada and Great Britain, for quite some time (Wachter & Goldman, 1996). Additionally, early in the continuum of care, speech-language pathologists may encounter critical care specialists or intensivists. Intensivists work exclusively in ICUs, with their primary goal to improve care and decrease mortality rates in ICUs (Kahn & Rubenfeld, 2015; Young & Birkmeyer, 2000).

During the early stage of medical care, the speech-language pathologist may encounter a radiologist, especially when working with patients with dysphagia. According to the American Board of Medical Specialties, radiologists are physicians specializing in different imaging techniques to diagnose and treat a variety of medical conditions (American Board of Medical Specialties [ABMS], 2018a, 2018b). Subspecialties within radiology include neuroradiology and pediatric radiology. Patients presenting with cancers or other diseases affecting the ears, nose, sinuses, face, jaw, and throat will be working with otolaryngologists. Otolaryngologists (or "ENTs") representing the Ear, Nose, and Throat specialty) are surgeons who specialize in diag-

nosing and treating these areas of the human body. Subspecialties may include neurotology, pediatrics, and plastic surgery. Board certification requires 5 years of residency (ABMS, 2018c). Throughout the continuum of care, the speech-language pathologist may also work closely with neurologists to determine the best care for patients with neurological disorders or diseases. Neurologists require four years of specialty training prior to board certification and focus on evaluating and treating conditions related to the central and peripheral nervous systems and their vascular supply. Subspecialties include brain injury and neurodevelopmental disabilities (ABMS, 2018a).

During the rehabilitation phase, speech-language pathologists will be closely working with physiatrists. Physiatrists are physicians with four years of specialty training and one year of clinical practice who concentrate on the evaluation and treatment of physical and cognitive impairments from musculoskeletal and neurological disorders. They work with the rehabilitation team to help patients with a variety of daily activities involving physical and cognitive functions (ABMS, 2018d). Speech-language pathologists working with older adults will encounter a geriatrician in some settings. Geriatricians are family physicians who specialize in geriatric medicine and have training targeting the aging process and illnesses in the older adult (ABMS, 2018a). Of course, on the other end of the life span are pediatricians who specialize in diagnosing and treating diseases found in children (birth to young adulthood age) (ABMS, 2018e). Speech-language pathologists also may work closely with psychiatrists. Psychiatrists specialize in diagnosing and treating mental and emotional disorders. Specialty training requires four years and subspecialties include child and adolescent psychiatry, as well as geriatric psychiatry (ABMS, 2018a).

Table 1–1. Examples of Different Physician Specialties and Their Area of Expertise

Physician Specialty	Primary Involvement	Examples of Potential Collaboration with Speech-Language Pathologists
Gynecology and Obstetrics	Treatment and diagnosis of diseases of the female reproductive system; branch of medicine and surgery concerned with childbirth	SLPs may receive referrals to support infants who have feeding/swallowing difficulty because of being born prematurely, or having muscle weakness, a cleft lip/palate, and so forth.
Hospitalist	Provides inpatient medicine	SLPs frequently receive consults from hospitalists to provide inpatient speech, language, cognitive, and swallowing services.
Neurology	Treatment and diagnosis of diseases of the nervous system	SLPs can provide critical information regarding speech and language to help neurologists reach a neurological diagnosis, such as Parkinson disease, myasthenia gravis, or primary progressive aphasia.
Nephrology	Treatment and diagnosis of disorders of the kidney	SLPs may receive a consult to support cognitive functioning or swallowing in a person with chronic renal failure.
Otolaryngology	Treatment and diagnosis of diseases of the ear, nose, and throat	SLPs receive referrals from otolaryngologists to help someone who had a mass from their vocal cords with a vocal fold pathology, or someone who would benefit from education regarding vocal hygiene.
Pediatrics	Specializes in treating and diagnosing diseases in children	SLPs may be asked to evaluate a child who is not reaching developmental milestones related to social communication, speech, language, literacy, and so forth.
Physiatry	Specializes in rehabilitative medicine	SLPs can be part of a rehabilitation team, along with the physiatrist, physical therapist, occupational therapist, and so forth, to support communication, cognition, and swallowing function in individuals with stroke or traumatic brain injury.
Plastic Surgery	Cosmetic and reconstructive surgery to change the body's appearance	SLPs may receive referrals to work with children with craniofacial anomalies who need numerous reconstructive surgeries.
Psychiatry[a]	Diagnosis and treatment (typically pharmacological) of mental health issues[a]	SLPs may be asked to work with a person who is experiencing negative side effects from neuroleptic medication, such as a person with schizophrenia who developed tardive dyskinesia (a movement disorder) that can affect speech and swallowing.

Table 1–1. *continued*

Physician Specialty	Primary Involvement	Examples of Potential Collaboration with Speech-Language Pathologists
Pulmonology	Treatment and diagnosis of diseases of the lungs	SLPs might work in tandem with a pulmonologist for people who have respiratory complications affecting their speech, such as people with amyotrophic lateral sclerosis, spinal cord injury, or multiple sclerosis.
Radiology	Uses imaging techniques to assess and treat health conditions	SLPs rely on radiologists to interpret imaging related to swallow function and brain scans.

Note. [a]Psychiatrists differ from psychologists, who focus extensively on psychotherapy and treating emotional and mental suffering using behavioral intervention (and are not permitted to prescribe medication in most states).

Physician's Assistants

Essential to the medical team are physician's assistants (Hooker & Everett, 2012). Physician assistants (PA) first emerged in the United States in 1967; currently, there are over 90,000 certified PAs, with a projection of over 43,000 primary care PAs in the United States by 2025 (Glicken & Miller, 2013; Hooker, 2006; Hooker, Cawley, & Everett, 2011). The PA is viewed as a health professional who collaborates, yet is supervised by, a physician in many different medical settings and specialties. Training for PAs is about 27 months, and different states have different licensure requirements.

Nurses

Nurses have been an important component of health care for centuries and the profession's contemporary manifestation is complex, diverse, and multifaceted. According to Black (2017), there are several different degree levels for nursing. For instance, the Bachelor's of Science in Nursing (BSN) degree is obtained after a four year university education, the Associate Degree in Nursing (ADN) requires a two year degree from a community college or technical school, or one can obtain a diploma in nursing from a hospital-based program. Additionally, nurses can acquire generalist and specialist certifications that prepare them to help patients in certain hospital units. There are also clinical nurse specialists (CNS) who have advanced degrees (master's, postmaster's, doctoral degrees) in specialty areas, clinical nurse leaders (CNL) who have master's level training, and advanced practice nurses (APN) who are registered nurses (RN) with more than a basic nursing education. Furthermore, there are nurse practitioners (NP) who have master's degrees or postmasters certificates who fulfill a semi-autonomous role alongside physicians, although this reliance differs from state to state (Black, 2017).

Other Medical Specialties

In addition to physicians and nurses, there are other specialists with whom medical speech-language pathologists frequently interact, including psychologists, neuropsychologists, social workers, and dieticians/clinical nutritionists. Psychologists assess and treat adults and children with mental and emotional problems, while focusing on behaviors influencing mental health. A subspecialty within psychology is rehabilitation psychology, which focuses on stroke, brain injury, developmental and intellectual disabilities and the personal adjustment, relations, and vocational issues related to these disabilities (American Psychological Association [APA], 2011). Another specialty of psychology is clinical neuropsychology. Neuropsychologists focus on brain-behavior relations through assessment and intervention associated with normal and abnormal function of the central nervous system. Neuropsychologists have a doctoral degree with further post-doctoral training (APA, 2010). Relatedly, social workers assist people with challenging life events (APA, 2010). According to the Bureau of Labor Statistics, as part of this assistance, social workers diagnose and treat issues related to mental, behavioral, and emotional health. Clinical social workers must have a master's degree and two years of postmaster's training (Bureau of Labor Statistics, 2018). Finally, registered dieticians (RD) are important colleagues for speech-language pathologists working with patients with dysphagia. Registered dietitians have completed an undergraduate degree, fulfilled an internship, passed a national examination, and are trained to manage all aspects of nutrition care, including screening, assessment/diagnosis, plan of care, and nutrition monitoring. They work in many different health care settings, including hospitals and long-term care facilities (Anderson et al., 2018). Dieticians and speech-language pathologists frequently work together to determine enteral and parenteral nutrition recommendations.

THE REHABILITATION TEAM

Speech-language pathologists are valuable members of a rehabilitation team consisting of physical therapists, occupational therapists, as well as respiratory therapists, music thera-

pists, and recreational therapists. The goal of this team is to facilitate the return of patients to their highest level of functioning. Over the years, the nomenclature describing the collaborative work between the disciplines has varied using terms such as multidisciplinary, interdisciplinary, and transdisciplinary, with all of these having different meanings and forms of interaction (Choi & Park, 2006). Perhaps the most current model is one utilizing a transdisciplinary approach integrating the different sciences and transcending traditional boundaries (Choi & Park, 2006). Despite what may be the existing popular trend, health professionals in the rehabilitation team maintain a consistent description of their primary roles and training requirements.

According to the American Physical Therapy Association (APTA), physical therapists (PT) assess and treat people across the lifespan to help in the areas of mobility and movement, pain management, improving function, reducing disability, and building healthy active lifestyles (American Physical Therapy Association [APTA], 2016). Graduates from physical therapy programs in 2018, and thereafter, must have a clinical doctorate degree (DPT). For those graduating from 2003 to 2017, there must be evidence of a postbaccalaureate degree in order to practice. Physical therapy providers who currently have a Bachelor's or Masters of Physical Therapy (graduating prior to 2003) can be licensed and practice in the United States. There are many postprofessional (transition) programs that provide training for physical therapists who hold the bachelor's and master's degrees, and would like to obtain the DPT. Physical therapy assistants (PTA) are supervised by PTs, carryout certain treatment components and may modify therapy according to the PT's recommendation. PTAs need a two-year associates degree, earned from an accredited training program. Most states do require a license or certification for employment (APTA, 2015).

Occupational therapists (OTs) assess and treat patients across the lifespan to foster participation in any desired daily activity by addressing cognition, psychology, and the physical abilities of an individual. By July 1, 2027, the entry-level degree requirement for OTs will be the professional doctorate degree; until then either a master's degree or professional doctorate in OT is required for employment. Similar to PTAs, occupational therapy assistants (OTA or COTA for certified OT assistant) carry out the treatment plan created by their supervising occupational therapist. The OTA is required to have a two-year associate's degree (The American Occupational Therapy Association, Inc., 2018).

As part of the rehabilitation team, certified respiratory therapists (CRT), or registered respiratory therapists (RRT) play an essential role in diagnosing and recommending treatments for lung and respiratory problems associated with disease or trauma, as well as managing ventilators and other airway tools for patients with respiratory difficulty (American Association for Respiratory Care [AARC], 2018a). The CRT has completed a two-year associate's degree, or a four-year bachelor's degree, followed by successful passing of a national examination. The RRT has a similar education background but has passed an additional national examination (AARC, 2018b).

The collaboration between music therapists and speech-language pathologists during the rehabilitation process is receiving greater attention and support (Laures-Gore, 2016). Music therapy is a health profession that uses music to address a wide range of social, physical, and cognitive disorders (American Music Therapy Association, 2018a). One of the great strengths of music therapy is that it can provide a means of communication for those who have difficulty expressing themselves through other modes. There are many paths outlined by the American Music Therapy Association for becoming a music therapist, however, the entry-level degree is a bachelor's degree (American Music Therapy Association, 2018b).

Recreational therapists are also a critical component of the rehabilitation team. To become a certified therapeutic recreation specialist (CTRS), one must have minimally a bachelor's degree, complete an internship, and pass a national examination (National Council for Therapeutic Recreation Certification [NCTRC], n.d.). Similar to other therapeutic professions, recreational therapists address many of the physical, cognitive, and emotional needs of patients, however, they also emphasize a patient's leisure needs. The leisure interests are incorporated into therapy, along with community resources to improve their daily living activities (American Therapeutic Recreation Association, 2018).

Finally, child life specialists (CLS) are essential to the medical care of children across different settings. These specialists utilize therapeutic play and education to help infants through adolescents and their families cope with the stressors associated with illnesses and injuries (Association of Child Life Professionals, 2018). To become a certified child life professional after 2019 (the year in which new requirements are implemented), one must complete a bachelor's degree with coursework in specific areas, a 600-hour internship, and a national examination. The American Academy of Pediatrics has published a policy statement regarding the importance of this field and its positive impact on children and families (Committee on Hospital Care and Child Life Council, 2014).

HEALTH ORGANIZATION STRUCTURE AND PROCESS

Medical settings often seek accreditation as a way to assure high quality of care for patients (Sack et al., 2011; Schmaltz, Williams, Chassin, Loeb, & Wachter, 2011). In the United

States, the Joint Commission (JC) is the primary accrediting agency for medical settings. There is also the Joint Commission International (JCI), an affiliate of the JC (Devkaran & O'Farrell, 2015). The aim of both commissions is to improve health care quality across many different settings. Health care organizations spend considerable resources on accreditation (Sack et al., 2011). The accreditation process involves an onsite visit and an evaluation of compliance with the JC standards. As of 2018, there were 20,000 health care organizations accredited by the JC and more than 1,000 accredited internationally (The Joint Commission [JC], 2018a; Joint Commission International, n.d.). Furthermore, the JC offers Disease Specific Care Certification in many different areas, including physical medicine/rehabilitation, cardiovascular, trauma, and neurology (JC, 2018b). A separate application and review process are required for successful certification.

Specific to rehabilitation, the Commission on Accreditation of Rehabilitation Facilities (CARF) is an international nonprofit organization that many rehabilitation and skilled nursing facilities seek out for accreditation. Successful accreditation from this agency involves multiple steps including a self-evaluation, application, and a site visit from a survey team (CARF International, 2018b). There are different levels of accreditation (3 year, 1 year, and provisional). Many facilities will seek out this accreditation because it symbolizes a commitment to quality patient care and demonstrates accountability to multiple stakeholders (CARF International, 2018a). Maintenance of accreditation requires facilities to submit an annual report.

Accurate and detailed clinical documentation within a health care setting is important for accreditation purposes, patient care, as well as reimbursement for medical services. Over the years, health care organizations have moved toward electronic health records (EHR) to summarize patient care, including clinical visits, therapy progress, and so on. These EHRs present in different forms across different settings, but often combine three elements: time orientation (temporal flow of information), source orientation (information per each team member), and problem orientation (Chaudhry et al., 2006; Häyrinen, Saranto, & Nykänen, 2008). Problem-oriented EHRs are encountered by many therapist; this element presents itself as the subjective, objective, assessment, plan (SOAP) notes. Speech-language pathologists in the medical setting use SOAP notes daily to summarize therapy sessions. All documentation should indicate the need for skilled services and the goals that were addressed during the therapy session. Accurate documentation is crucial as SOAP notes or other types of summaries will be read by other health professionals and used by payers to determine reimbursement.

An important aspect of documentation is coding. Codes are used as a means to communicate between speech-language pathology service providers and payers. ASHA (2018) provides a very thorough overview of the following three coding systems that speech-language pathologists use in the medical settings: the International Classification of Diseases, 10th Revision, Clinical Modification (ICD-10-CM); Current Procedural Terminology (CPT); and, the Healthcare Common Procedure Coding System (HCPCS). These three systems are used for different purposes (services vs. equipment) and for different reimbursers. Table 1–2 shows the differentiation of codes and examples of "each. Codes are occasionally updated and changed, so speech-language pathologists are required to be aware of the most current coding schema. In addition to the importance of coding for reimbursement, speech-language pathologists working in any medical setting need to be mindful of the

Table 1–2. Coding Systems and Examples of Common Codes

Coding System	Purpose	Examples	
International Classification of Diseases (ICD)	Diagnoses and procedures	F80.0	Developmental disorders related to speech and language
		I69.01	Cognitive deficits following nontraumatic subarachnoid hemorrhage
		I69.32	Speech and language deficits following cerebral infarction
		J38.2	Nodules of vocal cords
		P92	Feeding problems of newborns
		R13.1	Dysphagia
Current Procedural Terminology (CPT)	Procedures and services	92507	Treatment of speech, language, voice, communication, and/or auditory processing disorder, individual
		92521	Evaluation of speech fluency
		92522	Evaluation of speech sound production with evaluation of language comprehension and expression
Healthcare Common Procedure Coding System (HCPS)	Supplies, equipment, and devices, and procedures not in CPT	E2508	Speech generating device, synthesized speech, requiring message formulation by spelling and access by physical contact with the device
		L8500	Artificial larynx
		V5336	Repair/modification of augmentative communicative system or device (excludes adaptive hearing aid)

ASHA Sources: https://www.asha.org/Practice/reimbursement/coding/ICD-10/; https://www.asha.org/practice/reimbursement/coding/SLPCodeInfo/; https://www.asha.org/practice/reimbursement/coding/hcpcs_slp/

Health Insurance Portability and Accountability Act 1996 (HIPAA; Public Law 104-191). This act protects the privacy of patients among other purposes, including eliminating fraud and abuse by insurance companies. All health care providers must abide by this law and are restricted from sharing protected health information with other entities, including family members, unless otherwise indicated.

Payment for speech-language pathology services can occur through three primary mechanisms. Private pay is an individual paying for services out-of-pocket; the payment is directly from the consumer. The other two sources are private or public health insurers. There are many private insurers in the United States. Each company requires different types of documentation from service providers, and each has various qualifications for paying for services. In the 1990s, many private insurers became part of managed care that integrates all functions of health care delivery while controlling the price and utilization of services (Shi & Singh, 2014). There is evidence that managed care is beneficial, but may also have potential pitfalls (Gillian, David, David, & Flemming, 1997). Public health insurers include Medicare, Medicaid, and Children's Health Insurance Program (CHIP). Medicare is a federal program that serves people who are elderly and/or disabled. Medicaid, both federal- and state-funded, provides health care for people whose income is below a certain level (Shi & Singh, 2014). Similarly, CHIP is a federal/state-funded program serving children from low-income families (Shi & Singh, 2014). The process for providing speech-language services and reimbursement differs between the three public insurers.

CONCLUSION

The medical speech-language pathologist has many roles and responsibilities across wide-ranging health care environments. The collaboration between the medical speech-language pathologist and the myriad medical and rehabilitation team members is crucial for successful patient care. The health care environment is affected by federal and state laws and funding sources, thus, it is important for speech-language pathologists to remain informed about changing policies influencing their profession and patients.

REFERENCES

American Association of Critical-Care Nurses. (2009). *Progressive care fact sheet.* Retrieved from http://www.aacn.org/WD/Practice/Docs/ProgressiveCareFactSheet.pdf

American Association for Respiratory Care. (2018a). *What is an RT?* Retrieved from http://www.aarc.org/careers/what-is-an-rt/

American Association for Respiratory Care. (2018b). *Respiratory therapist credentials: CRT and RRT.* Retrieved from http://www.aarc.org/careers/how-to-become-an-rt/requirements/

American Board of Medical Specialties. (2018a). *ABMS guide to medical specialties.* Retrieved from http://www.abms.org/media/176512/abms-guide-to-medical-specialties-2018.pdf

American Board of Medical Specialties. (2018b). *American board of radiology.* Retrieved from http://www.abms.org/member-boards/contact-an-abms-memberboard/american-board-of-radiology/

American Board of Medical Specialties. (2018c). *American board of otolaryngology.* Retrieved from http://www.abms.org/member-boards/contact-an-abms-member-board/american-board-of-otolaryngology/

American Board of Medical Specialties. (2018d). *American board of physical medicine and rehabilitation.* Retrieved from http://www.abms.org/member-boards/contact-anabms-member-board/american-board-of-physical-medicine-and-rehabilitation/

American Board of Medical Specialties [ABMS]. (2018e). *American board of pediatrics.* Retrieved from http://www.abms.org/member-boards/contact-an-abms-member-board/american-board-of-pediatrics/

American Music Therapy Association. (2018a). *What is music therapy.* Retrieved from https://www.musictherapy.org/about/musictherapy/

American Music Therapy Association. (2018b). *Information for becoming a music therapist.* Retrieved from https://www.musictherapy.org/careers/information_for_becoming_a_music_therapist/

American Occupational Therapy Association, Inc. (2018). *American occupational therapy association, Inc. (AOTA).* Retrieved from https://www.aota.org/

American Physical Therapy Association. (2015). *Physical therapist assistant (PTA) education overview.* Retrieved from http://www.apta.org/PTAEducation/Overview/

American Physical Therapy Association. (2016). *Role of a physical therapist.* Retrieved from https://www.apta.org/PTCareers/RoleofaPT/

American Psychological Association. (2010). *Clinical neuropsychology.* Retrieved from http://www.apa.org/ed/graduate/specialize/neuro.aspx

American Psychological Association. (2011). *Careers in psychology.* Retrieved from http://www.apa.org/careers/resources/guides/careers.pdf

American Speech-Language-Hearing Association. (2016). *Scope of practice in speech language pathology.* Retrieved from http://www.asha.org/policy/

American Speech-Language-Hearing Association. (2018). *Billing and reimbursement.* Retrieved from https://www.asha.org/Practice/reimbursement/

American Therapeutic Recreation Association. (2018). *FAQ about RT/TR.* Retrieved from https://www.atra-online.com/what/FAQ

Anderson, D., Baird, S., Bates, T., Chapel, D. L., Cline, A. D., Ganesh, S. N., . . . McCauley, S. M. (2018). Academy of nutrition and dietetics: Revised 2017 standards of practice in nutrition care and standards of professional performance for registered dietitian nutritionists. *Journal of the Academy of Nutritional Dietetics, 118*(1), 132–140.

Association of American Medical Colleges. (2016). *2016 physician specialty data report.* Retrieved from https://www.aamc.org/data/workforce/reports/457712/2016specialtydatabook.html

Association of American Medical Colleges. (2018). *The road to becoming a doctor.* Retrieved from https://www.aamc.org/download/68806/data/road-doctor.pdf

Association of Child Life Professionals. (2018). *Mission, values, vision.* Retrieved from https://www.childlife.org/child-life-profession/mission-values-vision

Balanced Budget Act, Pub. L. No. 105-33, 111 Stat 251 (1997).

Black, B. (2017). *Professional nursing: Concepts and challenges* (8th ed.). St. Louis, MO: Elsevier.

Bureau of Labor Statistics. (2018). *Occupational outlook handbook: Social workers.* Retrieved from https://www.bls.gov/ooh/community-and-social-service/mobile/social-workers.htm

CARF International. (2018a). *Accreditation benefits.* Retrieved from http://www.carf.org/Accreditation/ValueOfAccreditation/Benefits/

CARF International. (2018b). *Steps to accreditation.* Retrieved from http://www.carf.org/Accreditation/AccreditationProcess/StepstoAccreditation/

Chaudhry, B., Wang, J., Wu, S., Maglione, M., Mojica, W., Roth, E., . . . Shekelle, P. G. (2006). Systematic review: Impact of health information technology on quality, efficiency, and costs of medical care. *Annals of Internal Medicine, 144*(10), 742–752.

Choi, B. C., & Pak, A. W. (2006). Multidisciplinarity, interdisciplinarity and transdisciplinarity in health research, services, education and policy: 1. Definitions, objectives, and evidence of effectiveness. *Clinical and Investigative Medicine, 29*(6), 351.

Committee on Hospital Care and Child Life Council. (2014). Policy statement: Child life services. *Pediatrics, 133*(5), e1471–e1478.

Devkaran, S., & O'Farrell, P. N. (2015). The impact of hospital accreditation on quality measures: An interrupted time series analysis. *BMC Health Services Research, 15,* 137. http://doi.org/10.1186/s12913-015-0784-5

Freidson, E. (1970). *Professional dominance: The social structure of medical care.* Chicago, IL: Aldine.

Gillian, F., David, J. H., David, M., & Flemming, R. (1997). Managed care: Implications of managed care for health systems, clinicians, and patients. *British Medical Journal, 314.* https://doi.org/10.1136/bmj.314.7098.1895

Glicken, A. D., & Miller, A. A. (2013). Physician assistants: From pipeline to practice. *Academic Medicine, 88*(12), 1883–1889.

Häyrinen, K., Saranto, K., & Nykänen, P. (2008). Definition, structure, content, use and impacts of electronic health records: A review of the research literature. *International Journal of Medical Informatics, 77,* 291–304.

Health Insurance Portability and Accountability Act of 1996, Pub. L. No. 104–191, 110 Stat. 1938 (1996).

Hooker, R. S. (2006). Physician assistants and nurse practitioners: The United States experience. *Medical Journal of Australia, 185*(1), 4.

Hooker, R. S., Cawley, J. F., & Everett, C. M. (2011). Predictive modeling the physician assistant supply: 2010–2025. *Public Health Reports, 126*(5), 708–716.

Hooker, R. S., & Everett, C. M. (2012). The contribution of physician assistants in primary care systems. *Health and Social Care in the Community, 20*(1), 20–31. http://doi.org/10.1111/j.1365-2524.2011.01021.x

The Joint Commission. (2018a). *About the Joint Commission.* Retrieved from https://www.joint commission.org/about_us/about_the_joint_commission_main.aspx

The Joint Commission. (2018b). *Disease specific care certification.* Retrieved from https://www.jointcommission.org/certification/dsc_home.aspx

Joint Commission International. (n.d.). *JCI-Accredited organizations.* Retrieved from https://www.jointcommissioninternational.org/about-jci/jci-accredited-organizations/

Kahn, J. M., & Rubenfeld, G. D. (2015). The myth of the workforce crisis. Why the United States does not need more intensivist physicians. *American Journal of Respiratory and Critical Care Medicine, 191*(2), 128–134.

Landrigan, C. P., Conway, P. H., Edwards, S., & Srivastava, R. (2006). Pediatric hospitalists: A systematic review of the literature. *Pediatrics, 117*(5), 1736–1744.

Laures-Gore, J. (2016). Perspectives: The humanities and speech-language pathology. *Journal of Humanities in Rehabilitation.* Retrieved from https://scholarblogs.emory.edu/journalofhumanitiesinrehabilitation/2016/11/30/perspectives-the-humanities-and-speech-language-pathology-in-rehabilitation/

National Council for Therapeutic Recreation Certification. (n.d.). *Certification standards.* Retrieved from https://nctrc.org/about-certification/certification-standards/

National Institute on Deafness and Other Communication Disorders. (2016, May 19). *Quick statistics about voice, speech, language.* Retrieved from https://www.nidcd.nih.gov/health/statistics/quick-statistics-voice-speech-language#ftn1

Patient Protection and Affordable Care Act, 42 U.S.C. § 18001 (2010).

Prin, M., & Wunsch, H. (2014). The role of stepdown beds in hospital care. *American Journal of Respiratory and Critical Care Medicine, 190*(11). https://doi.org/10.1164/rccm.2014061117PP

Rachoin, J. S., Skaf, J., Cerceo, E., Fitzpatrick, E., Milcarek, B., Kupersmith, E., & Scheurer, D. B. (2012). The impact of hospitalists on length of stay and costs: Systematic review and meta-analysis. *American Journal of Managed Care, 18*(1), 23–30.

Robinson, J. H., Callister, L. C., Berry, J. A., & Dearing, K. A. (2008), Patient-centered care and adherence: Definitions and applications to improve outcomes. *Journal of the American Academy of Nurse Practitioners, 20,* 600–607.

Sack C., Scherag, A., Lütkes, P., Günther, W., Jöckel K. H., & Holtmann G. (2011). Is there an association between hospital accreditation and patient satisfaction with hospital care? A survey of 37, 000 patients treated by 73 hospitals. *International Journal for Quality in Health Care, 23*(3), 278–283. https://doi.org/10.1093/intqhc/mzr011

Schmaltz, S. P., Williams, S. C., Chassin, M. R., Loeb, J. M., & Wachter, R. M. (2011). Hospital performance trends on national quality measures and the association with Joint Commission accreditation. *Journal of Hospital Medicine, 6*(8), 454–461. https://doi.org/10.1002/jhm.905

Shi, L., & Singh, D. A. (2014). *Delivering health care in America: A systems approach* (6th ed.). Burlington, MA: Jones & Bartlett Learning.

Stacy, K. M. (2011). Progressive care units: Different but the same. *Critical Care Nurse, 31*(3), 77–81. https://doi.org/10.4037/ccn2011644

Wachter, R. M., & Goldman, L. (1996). The emerging role of "hospitalists" in the American health care system. *New England Journal of Medicine, 335,* 514–517.

Wachter, R. M., & Goldman, L. (2016). Zero to 50,000—the 20th anniversary of the hospitalist. *New England Journal of Medicine, 375*(11), 1009–1011.

World Health Organization. (2001). *International classification of functioning, disability and health: ICF.* Geneva, Switzerland: Author.

Young, M. P., & Birkmeyer, J. D. (2000). Potential reduction in mortality rates using an intensivist model to manage intensive care units. *Effective Clinical Practice: ECP, 3*(6), 284–289.

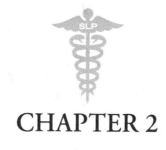

CHAPTER 2

Clinical Populations Encountered by the Medical Speech-Language Pathologist

Rene Ruzicka Kanadet, Doreen Kelly Izaguirre,
Matina Balou, and Kristie A. Spencer

INTRODUCTION

Kristie A. Spencer

The medical speech-language pathologist (SLP) can work in a wide variety of settings, spanning general medical facilities, Veterans Affairs medical centers, long-term acute care hospitals, rehabilitation hospitals, pediatric hospitals, neonatal intensive care units, skilled nursing facilities, home health agencies, and outpatient clinics. Given this vast range of settings, the clinical populations encountered by a medical SLP are remarkably diverse. The standard caseload of a medical SLP may be influenced by the particular setting or the particular unit within a medical facility (e.g., a brain injury unit). According to a recent survey by the American Speech-Language Hearing Association (ASHA, 2017), the most common areas of intervention for an SLP will differ depending on the type of facility in which the SLP works. For example, time spent on aphasia and traumatic brain injury was highest among SLPs in outpatient clinics or rehabilitation hospitals, whereas time spent on dementia was highest in skilled nursing facilities. Time spent on swallowing was highest in general medical facilities and hospitals, whereas time spent on augmentative and alternative communication was highest for SLPs in the home health arena. Despite the overall trends, SLPs in these settings continue to encounter individuals with a wide variety of diagnoses. Most medical SLPs will need to be generalists and prepared to serve anyone in the medical setting who faces communication or swallowing challenges. Consequently, medical SLPs need specialty knowledge in areas such as anatomy and physiology, neural control of movement, medication effects, neuroimaging, and infection control. They will often encounter patients with primary and secondary diagnoses, and will be challenged to understand how these diagnoses interact. For example, in a hospital, the medical SLP might work with an adult with a recent acquired brain injury from a fall who also has a developmental disorder, such as cerebral palsy.

This chapter is intended to provide a sampling of the varied clinical populations with which a medical SLP may interact. The populations summarized here are intended to represent patients from a wide range of health care settings and include individuals with developmental disorders, acquired brain injuries, neurodegenerative disorders, encephalopathies, psychiatric disorders, cardiac and respiratory disorders, head and neck surgeries, and esophageal disorders.

DEVELOPMENTAL DISORDERS

Rene Ruzicka Kanadet

Developmental disorders provide a particular challenge to the hospital speech-language pathologist. Pediatric SLPs are well versed in the cognitive-communication, language, speech, and swallowing difficulties faced by children with developmental disorders; however, these children grow into adults and are hospitalized for a variety of reasons. The hospital clinician may be asked to do an evaluation and must consider the baseline functioning of these individuals. It also must be kept in mind that new medical issues, superimposed on baseline dysphagia, dysarthria, and cognitive-communication impairments, may result in exacerbated deficits and/or may not present as expected for new diagnoses. For example, speech following a focal cortical stroke may be a mixed dysarthria due to the patient's baseline developmental dysarthria. Although there are many to consider, a few major diagnoses are highlighted here.

Cerebral Palsy and Muscular Dystrophy

Cerebral palsy and muscular dystrophy are common pediatric disorders that affect movement, though their cause, presentation, and progression are quite different. What they have in common is that speech production and swallowing may be impacted, and intellectual impairments are possible with certain subtypes of the disorders.

Nature of Cerebral Palsy

Cerebral palsy (CP) is caused by abnormal development of the brain in a fetus or by damage to the brain during or shortly after birth. This damage may be secondary to intracranial hemorrhage or hypoxic-ischemic encephalopathy. There are multiple types of CP, including ataxic, dyskinetic, spastic, and mixed. Spastic is the most common, and there are three types: spastic hemiplegia/hemiparesis, spastic diplegia/diparesis, and spastic quadriplegia/quadriparesis. CP is not a progressive disorder; however, the presentation of specific symptoms may change across the lifespan, and the effects of aging may be evident in young adults with CP (Haak, Lenski, Hidecker, Li, & Paneth, 2009).

Potential Impact on Communication/Swallowing

Impairments in speech and swallowing are related to motor coordination and control. There is variability in presentation based on the type and severity of CP. Cited dysarthria types include spastic, ataxic, and hyperkinetic (Schölderle, Staiger, Lampe, & Ziegler, 2013). Persons with spastic quadriplegia/quadriparesis are more likely to present with severe dysarthria and may be nonverbal, requiring AAC. Cognitive-communication impairments are most common with this type of CP as well (Fennell & Dikel, 2001). Presence of epilepsy is also linked with mental retardation in individuals with CP (Venkateswaran & Shevell, 2008).

There are high rates of dysphagia in the CP population (Salghetti & Martinuzzi,

2012). Characteristics include anterior loss of material, tongue thrust, poor oral control, oral residue, delayed trigger of the pharyngeal swallow, and multiple swallows (Menezes, Santos, & Alves, 2017). Additional clinical observations may include facial grimacing, head tilt, and prolonged meal times. Discoordination of respiration and deglutition may be seen, with possible stridor, coughing, and apnea during meals resulting in increased aspiration risk. Additional complicating factors may include difficulty with self-feeding due to reduced motor control, uncontrolled body movements during feeding/swallowing, and position. Despite these factors, many people with CP learn to compensate and are very functional eaters throughout their lifetime.

Nature of Muscular Dystrophy

Muscular dystrophy (MD) represents a group of several heterogeneous disorders characterized by progressive muscle weakness (Mercuri & Muntoni, 2013). There are multiple types of MD, though they do not all affect speech and swallowing. The most well known is Duchenne MD, characterized by progressive muscle weakness beginning with the pelvis and arms, and eventually spreading to all voluntary muscles. Becker MD presents with the same symptoms as Duchenne MD, though it is less severe, progresses more slowly, and does not present until adolescence or early adulthood (Emery, 2002). Myotonic MD does not present until adulthood and may progress slowly for as long as 50 to 60 years. Symptoms include weakness and slow relaxation of muscles after contraction (De Swart, van Engelen, van De Kerkhof, & Maassen, 2004). Fascioscapulohumeral MD is characterized by weakness of the face, shoulder, and upper arm muscles, with an onset as early as infancy and as late as adulthood. The face, feet, hands, and neck are affected first. Oculopharyngeal MD presents in middle age and affects muscles of the eyelids and

pharynx with dysphagia as a primary symptom (Ruegg et al., 2005). Limb-girdle MD is characterized by weakness of upper and lower limbs, as well as pelvic-girdle weakness. Respiratory deficiencies may be present. Emery-Dreifuss MD typically presents by age 10 and is characterized by weakness of the shoulders, upper arms, and calf muscles, as well as cardiac problems. Congenital MD is unlikely to be seen by hospital SLPs who do not work with pediatrics, as lifespan is much shorter.

Potential Impact on Communication/Swallowing

Due to the variable onset of different MD types, not all Muscular Dystrophies can be considered developmental. As a hospital SLP, there may be patients who have lived with the progressive changes of MD for the majority of their lives, and there may be patients dealing with a very new diagnosis. The presence of dysphagia and dysarthria are dependent on which muscles have been impacted. Pharyngeal residue is a commonly cited problem for those with MD, as muscle weakness negatively impacts pharyngeal clearance (van den Engel-Hoek et al., 2013). Reduced respiratory support may lead to decreased coordination of respiration and swallowing and/or a weak cough that cannot sufficiently clear the airway. Facial and lingual weakness may cause oral phase problems, as well as dysarthria. Flaccid dysarthia is the most likely, with reduced articulatory precision related to lingual weakness, hypernasality resulting from palatal weakness, and decreased vocal intensity secondary to weak respiratory muscles (De Swart, et al., 2004; Duffy, 2013). Due to the slow progression, it is possible that patients with dysphagia will not report the symptoms, as they may have naturally learned to compensate. It is important to complete instrumental assessments, such as a videofluoroscopic swallow study (VFSS) and flexible endoscopic evaluation of swallowing (FEES), to assess current functioning and provide the best recommendations for safety.

Role of the SLP

For both muscular dystrophy and cerebral palsy, the hospital speech-language pathologist faces some challenges. The first is to determine baseline functioning prior to the hospitalization. Depending on the reason for admission, speech and swallowing skills may remain at baseline or be exacerbated by generalized weakness related to disease or hospitalization. To determine baseline, asking questions about dysphagia symptoms, home diet, and intelligibility are warranted. Asking the patient about changes to their speech and swallowing is informative; however, specific questions may be needed to gain greater insight. Consider the questions below.

- Do you avoid any foods, like nuts or corn?
- Tell me what you like to eat for breakfast (lunch/dinner)?
- Have you ever received the Heimlich maneuver?
- Do you ever feel like food is sticking in your throat or you need to drink water to help it go down?
- Are you a fast or slow eater?
- Do people ever ask you to repeat yourself? How often?
- Are you able to communicate on the phone?

Patients who have a long history of dysphagia, for example, those with CP, may be quick to minimize their current difficulty. It behooves the hospital SLP to follow clinical signs and complete assessments and treatments as appropriate, regardless of the concern expressed by the patient. For patients with MD, the hospital SLP may be the first to identify dysphagia. Education and compensatory training will be key roles of the hospital SLP during an acute admission. Referring to rehabilitation may also be appropriate. When dysarthria is severe or the person is nonverbal, it becomes necessary for the evaluating SLP to provide communication supports (e.g., picture/alphabet boards, determining reliable yes/no method) and to educate staff on the best ways to communicate with the patient (see Yorkston, Beukelman, Strand, & Hakel, 2010).

Down Syndrome

Nature of Down Syndrome

Down syndrome is a genetic disorder caused by the presence of an extra 21st chromosome. According to the Centers for Disease Control [CDC] (2017), approximately 1 in 700 children are born with Down syndrome in the United States. The clinical manifestations include distinct facial features, hypotonia, dysphagia, dysarthria, and intellectual disabilities, as well as additional medical issues, such as congenital heart disease. As with CP and other developmental diagnoses, it is important to determine the patient's baseline functioning. Family interview is the best route, if possible. Adults with Down syndrome may not be able to accurately report their baseline skills nor the level of assist that they require. Severity of deficits is variable, with some adults with Down syndrome being relatively high functioning, holding entry level jobs and living independently with some assistance, whereas others may be nonverbal and/or require full time care.

Life expectancy for persons with Down syndrome has increased significantly over the last 3 to 4 decades. In 1970, the life expectancy was 12 years old, whereas in 2007, it had increased to age 47 (CDC, 2017). Adults with Down syndrome are at higher risk for medical conditions including cancer, obesity, and dementia (Nixon, 2018), as well as adult-onset seizures, visual changes, and hearing loss (Esbensen, 2010). Hospitalization may occur for any of these conditions.

Potential Impact on Communication/Swallowing

Persons with Down syndrome often have an oral dysphagia related to low muscle tone, a tongue-thrust swallow pattern, and decreased oral-sensory awareness. These issues can lead to a messy appearance while eating, with poor bolus cohesion, disorganized lingual movement during mastication, oral residue, and at times, anterior loss of material before or during the swallow. There is also an increased risk for silent aspiration. A study from the Children's Hospital of Colorado revealed that most children with Down syndrome who received dysphagia imaging studies (i.e., VFSS or FEES) and were aspirating, did so silently (Jackson, Maybee, Moran, Wolter-Warmerdam, & Hickey, 2016).

Persons with Down syndrome often present with dysarthria, most likely the flaccid type, along with interdentalization of some sounds (e.g., /s/) related to tongue thrust. Severity is variable. Dysarthria, like dysphagia, may be exacerbated with generalized weakness, deconditioning, and/or a new diagnosis that can cause dysarthria. Treatment may target strategy use and/or providing communication supports, such as communication boards. Stuttering and/or cluttering occur at rates of 10% to 45%, compared with about 1% in the general population (Kent & Vorperian, 2013).

Role of the SLP

Formal assessment and treatment of cognitive-communication skills may not be appropriate.

Tests for these skills are not normed on a population with developmental intellectual disabilities, thereby limiting assessment options. Orientation tests, such as the Saint Louis University Mental Status Exam (SLUMS; Tariq, Tumosa, Chibnall, Perry, & Morley, 2006) or Orientation Log (Novack, 2000), may be used to monitor mental status changes across time. It may be useful to know the person's previous independence levels to determine if any intervention is appropriate. For example, for a person with Down syndrome who receives supervision during all activities of daily living (ADLs) and has a guardian who takes care of scheduling appointments, managing finances, and making medical decisions, cognitive treatment may not be warranted. Determining yes/no reliability and providing education to staff regarding communication strategies will be important. Although there is positive evidence regarding treatment of speech intelligibility in children with Down syndrome (Yoder, Camarata, & Woynaroski, 2016), assessment and treatment may not be a priority for a hospitalized adult and his/her family. For an adult with Down syndrome, the hospital SLP should be aware that signs of oral dysphagia on a clinical exam should be expected, and may be the person's baseline. It is important to ask the patient and family what types of foods that person typically eats at home. Ask specific questions about food and preparation to gain an accurate picture of the person's home diet. Despite the knowledge that the patient has a baseline dysphagia, it is imperative that clinical decision-making relates to the person's current symptoms and appropriate tests are completed if warranted. Consider that a person with a baseline dysphagia may be at even greater risk for aspiration when deconditioned or presenting with a new illness.

Another primary role of the hospital SLP will be advocacy. As discussed with other developmental diagnoses, it will be important to ensure that communication with the patient with Down syndrome is at an appropriate cognitive level to maximize understanding. The use of pictures, rate of instruction, and amount of information discussed will be important. It should also be determined early on if the person has a parent, sibling, or other family member who serves as a guardian and medical decision maker.

Autism

Nature of Autism

Autism spectrum disorder (ASD) refers to a group of diagnoses characterized by social communication impairments; speech/language impairments; restricted repetitive and stereotyped patterns of behavior, activities, and interests; sensory processing impairments; and executive function impairments (Pratt, Hopf, & Larriba-Quest, 2017). As suggested by the term spectrum, presence and severity of characteristics varies widely within the population and over time.

Potential Impact on Communication/Swallowing and Role of the SLP

The nature of the hospital environment may be very challenging or overwhelming to a person with ASD. For those with sensory processing difficulty, the fluorescent hospital lights, incessant beeping of machines, and busy, often loud environment may be extremely over-stimulating. Consider modifying the environment to optimize the person's participation and functioning. Closing doors, lowering lights, and providing a weighted blanket are all small actions that can make a big difference. When the person is higher functioning, they may be able to tell you what helps them. Otherwise, family report or allowing the family to alter the environment or provide supports is important.

Additionally, being in the hospital is outside of a person's routine and is often very unpredictable. Executive function deficits in persons with ASD include rigid, inflexible thinking. Many persons with ASD are distressed by changes to routine or schedules. Be aware that the patient may not be able or willing to engage or comply with requests on the timeline of the medical professional. It may be beneficial to provide the person with a schedule or plan to help them feel organized and understand what to expect. Visual supports can facilitate better understanding than auditory information, considering both attentional and language impairments that may exist. Utilizing pictures or written information can be very beneficial.

Pragmatic language deficits may include reduced eye contact, inappropriate statements, or decreased reciprocity during conversational exchanges. Expressive and/or receptive language may be impaired. Echolalia is one manifestation of a language impairment, characterized by immediate or delayed repetition of dialogue. This provides a challenge for medical professionals, as repetition of a statement is often used as acknowledgment of understanding and cannot be considered reliable for individuals demonstrating echolalia. Persons with more severe ASD may be nonverbal and have severe intellectual disabilities. The hospital SLP should provide communication and/or executive function supports for all individuals with ASD and educate medical staff on the best way to interact with the patient.

Dysphagia is not considered a typical characteristic of ASD; however, many persons with ASD eat a highly restricted diet. Schreck, Williams, and Smith (2004) reported that 72% of their study participants had restricted diets and more than 50% were reported to refuse foods. This is related to both the tendency for restricted, repetitive behaviors manifested in what and when the person will eat, as well as sensory processing impairments leading to refusal/avoidance of specific tastes, colors, and textures of foods. Persons with ASD may also be on a gluten- or casein-free diet, as some there is a belief that that this improves gastrointestinal symptoms and/or behavior, though limited conclusive evidence exists (Mulloy et al., 2009). The hospital SLP will be challenged to perform a clinical swallow evaluation if the patient is unwilling to accept the foods/liquids presented for testing. Responses to new foods/liquids may include refusal, distress, and/or gagging.

Further, some persons with ASD who have an extremely restricted diet may not have the oral motor skills to safely consume all consistencies. For example, if an individual only accepts liquids, he/she may not have developed skills for mastication. It is recommended that the evaluating SLP complete a brief clinical interview prior to presenting foods/liquids, asking questions specifically about the person's home diet. SLPs should also inquire about what types of cups, utensils, and other feeding tools are used by the patient, as some persons with ASD will not accept a new presentation. The most successful evaluation of skill will utilize familiar utensils/tools and preferred foods/liquids. These factors should also be considered prior to attempting an instrumental evaluation. If able to tolerate the procedure, a FEES would allow use of preferred foods/liquids. When a VFSS is necessary, introducing the barium products prior to evaluation may allow the patient to become familiar and accepting of the products. It can also identify patients who will absolutely not tolerate barium before going through the process of scheduling the assessment and transporting the patient to x-ray.

When reviewing a patient's medical history, consideration for developmental disorders is important. The outlook and priorities of the patient and family may differ significantly from a neurotypical adult. Case history with the patient and their family is imperative in

these cases to have a thorough understanding of prehospitalization functioning and responsibilities, home diet, caregiver assistance, and previous speech therapy participation. When assessment and/or treatment are not warranted, as the patient is performing at baseline, the SLP must consider their role as a patient advocate and educator to hospital staff who may be less familiar with appropriate communication, cognitive, and swallow strategies.

ACQUIRED BRAIN INJURY

Rene Ruzicka Kanadet with Kristie A. Spencer

Acquired brain injury refers to an acute injury to the brain, and includes stroke, traumatic brain injury, brain tumors, and anoxic/hypoxic brain injury. The clinical manifestations are variable and highly dependent upon the location and extent of the injury. Stroke and traumatic brain injury are highlighted here. A solid understanding of neuroanatomy is important for medical SLPs who work in hospital settings, especially trauma centers, certified stroke centers, and rehabilitation units.

Stroke

Description of Medical Condition

Stroke, also known as a cerebrovascular accident (CVA), occurs when there is sudden death of brain tissue secondary to a lack of blood and oxygen to an area of the brain. It can affect the cerebral cortex or subcortical structures. Strokes are differentiated by their cause: ischemic or hemorrhagic. An ischemic stroke, which is the most common and responsible for 87% of strokes, is caused by lack of oxygen to a region of the brain due to a blockage of blood flow to the brain (American Heart

Association, 2018a). Ischemic strokes are further classified as thrombotic (a blood clot develops within the blood vessel) or embolic (the blood clot or plaque originates elsewhere in the body and travels to the blood vessel in the brain). A hemorrhagic stroke is caused by bleeding into or around the brain, typically from a weakened blood vessel or an aneurysm. Initial symptoms may include numbness or weakness on one side of the body, difficulty walking, facial droop, changes to speech, vision changes, headache, and confusion. Stroke is confirmed through neuroimaging, including CT and MRI (American Heart Association, 2018b). When identified within a three-hour timeframe, tissue plasminogen activator (tPA) can be administered in the emergency room to slow stroke progression (Cheng & Kim, 2015). Risk factors for stroke include high blood pressure, high cholesterol, chronic kidney disease, smoking/tobacco use, inactivity, diabetes mellitus, disorders of heart rhythm, sleep apnea, and family history (Mozzaffarian et al., 2016).

Potential Impact on Communication/Swallowing

Strokes can cause a wide range of impairments, including disruption to language, cognition, and speech. Aphasia is an acquired language disorder that is present in 20% to 38% of individuals with stroke (Dickey et al., 2010), in most cases when the lesion is on the left, language-dominant side of the brain. Aphasia is classically described via the connectionist model as nonfluent (e.g., agrammatic verbal output) or fluent (e.g., grammatical speech with preserved prosody, but disrupted meaning). Hillis (2007) describes these classic nonfluent and fluent aphasia types and their corresponding lesion sites, such as Broca's aphasia, Wernicke's aphasia, and conduction aphasia. Though often used in medical settings (Yourganov, Smith, Fridriksson, & Rorden, 2015), the classical aphasia types can be misleading because they do not adequately describe the linguistic details of the language impairment and there is considerable variability as well as overlap across types. For instance, people with the same aphasia type can have different deficits, and identical deficits (e.g., anomia) can occur across different types. Another dichotomy that is still seen in many medical facilities is expressive aphasia (i.e., the patient has difficulty with expressive language) and receptive aphasia (i.e., the patient has difficulty comprehending), though these terms are misleading because patients with aphasia will have difficulty with both expression and comprehension along a continuum of dysfunction. Current conceptualizations of aphasia promote description of linguistic phenomena, such as semantics, syntax, and phonology (both receptively and expressively) when characterizing the patient's aphasia.

Cognitive-communication skills can also affected by stroke, particularly following multiple strokes and bilateral damage. Neuroanatomical lesions in areas such as the hippocampus and white matter lesions, as well as cerebral microbleeds due to cerebrovascular diseases, contribute to the pathogenesis of poststroke cognitive impairment (Sun, Tan, & Yu, 2014). Disruption can occur across cognitive domains, including attention, executive functions, memory, working memory, and processing speed (Cummings, Marshall, & Lazar, 2013). Right hemisphere lesions also commonly result in a constellation of cognitive-communication deficits, such as anosognosia (impaired awareness of deficits), hemispatial neglect, disrupted attention, and visuospatial impairment.

There is a high prevalence of dysphagia following acute stroke, with reports of 50% or greater (Mann, Hankey, & Cameron, 2000; Martino et al., 2005). Increased risk of dysphagia has been reported in patients with pontine, lateral medullary, and medial medullary lesions (Flowers, Skoretz, Streiner, Silver, & Martino, 2011). Additionally, Suntrup and colleagues (2015) reported that 82.5% of their study sample presented with dysphagia and determined that distinct brain lesion locations were related to the incidence, severity, and pattern of dysphagia. That is, lesion size was predictive of dysphagia, as was location with primary and secondary sensorimotor cortex; white matter pathways, such as the superior longitudinal fasciculus and corticospinal tract; descending cortical-bulbar fibers; temporal regions; and supramarginal gyrus associated with dysphagia. The supramarginal gyrus was the only area predictive of severe dysphagia in this sample (Suntrup et al., 2015). The study supported previous reports of left side stroke leading to greater oral phase deficits and right side stroke resulting in more pharyngeal deficits (Robbins, Levine, Maser, Rosenbek, & Kempster, 1993). Similarly, Hamdy et al. (1999) found through fMRI that cortical control of swallowing is bilateral but asymmetric, with a dominant hemisphere that does not correlate with handedness.

Motor speech disorders are also common following stroke. Flaccid or spastic dysarthria can occur following a stroke to the brainstem; spastic dysarthria may also emerge following disruption to the upper motor neurons bilaterally. Ataxic dysarthria may occur following a lesion to the cerebellar control circuit. Other forms of dysarthria, such as hypokinetic and hyperkinetic, are possible, but much less common, following stroke (Spencer & Brown, 2018). Stroke is the predominate cause of unilateral upper motor neuron (UUMN) dysarthria, which is associated with contralateral central face and tongue weakness (Duffy, 2013). Left carotid or middle cerebral artery occlusions can lead to a UUMN dysarthria, with likely concomitant aphasia or apraxia of speech. Right carotid or middle cerebral artery occlusions can also lead to a UUMN dysarthria, often with concomitant cognitive-communication impairment, such as visuospatial neglect or pragmatic deficits (Spencer & Brown, 2018). Regardless of dysarthria type, common descriptors of poststroke dysarthria include imprecise articulation and slow speaking rate, as well as possible voice changes, disrupted prosody, and altered respiratory control or coordination (Mackenzie, 2011). Apraxia of speech can also occur following a stroke; it reflects disruption to motor speech planning or programming. Lesion locations can vary, but recent research suggests a focus on the left premotor cortex and adjacent precentral gyrus (Graff-Radford et al., 2014). The key diagnostic characteristics of apraxia of speech include slow speech rate, disrupted prosody (equalized stress patterns, segregated character), and distorted sound errors.

Traumatic Brain Injury

Description of Medical Condition

A traumatic brain injury (TBI) refers to damage to the brain following some form of trauma. It is estimated that between 1.7 to 2.5 million people sustain a TBI each year in the United States (Faul, Xu, Wald, & Coronado, 2010; Brain Injury Association of America, 2018) with 1.1 to 1.3 million emergency department visits annually (Centers for Disease Control, 2010; Heegard & Biros, 2007). Sixty-nine million individuals worldwide are estimated to sustain a TBI each year (Dewan et al., 2018). The Brain Injury Association of America (2018) reports that falls are responsible for approximately 40% of diagnosed TBIs, with additional leading causes including motor vehicle accidents, being struck by or against something, and assault. Blast injuries from improvised explosive devices (IEDs) are a primary cause of brain injuries in the military population, and TBI is considered the signature injury of Operations Iraqi Freedom and Enduring Freedom (Farmer et al., 2017). Up to 20% of service members are estimated to experience a TBI (Farmer et al. 2017). While the majority of these injuries are classified as mild (Salat, Robinson, Miller, Clark, & McGlinchey, 2017), the sequelae of the brain injury can be markedly disruptive to day-to-day functioning. TBIs can be broadly classified as open head injuries that penetrate the meninges (three membranes that line the skull) and closed head injuries that do not penetrate the meninges. Severity of TBI is highly variable, ranging from concussion without loss of consciousness to severe injury and coma. The Glasgow Coma Scale (GCS) is often used to categorize the level of consciousness in an individual with TBI, based on motor responsiveness, verbal performance, and eye opening (Teasedale & Jennett, 1974). Patients receive a score between 3 to 15 and are categorized as severe (GCS <8), moderate (GCS 9 to 13), or mild (GCS 14 to 15). The Rancho Los Amigos Levels of Cognitive Functioning (Hagen, 2000) is also used to communicate the stage of recovery following TBI. The eight levels capture recovery indices such as the patient's response to the environment, level of confusion/agitation, degree of orientation, and type of assistance needed to complete activities of daily living.

When the skull hits an object, such as a dashboard or wall, there are several mechanisms of brain injury. Damage at the point of contact is referred to as the coup. Due to the brain's movement within the skull, damage also frequently occurs opposite to the point of contact, known as contracoup. Because the brain shifts rapidly within the skull, diffuse axonal injury (DAI) can occur, reflecting the disconnection or alteration of axons. DAI primarily affects the white matter tracts in the brain. It can lead to immediate and persistent coma. The presence of DAI in patients with TBI results in a higher chance of an unfavorable outcome, particularly with lesions in the corpus callosum (van Eijck, Schoonman, van der Naalt, de Vries, & Roks, 2018).

Secondary brain insults can also occur and stem from the destructive intracellular and extracellular pathologic processes that begin at the time of a TBI (Heegaard & Biros, 2007). For example, cerebral edema and increased intracranial pressure are common after a TBI and can lead to ischemia (Ghajar, 2000). Infections and seizures can also occur. Systemic insults include hypotension, hypo- and hypercapnia (reduced/excessive carbon dioxide in the blood), anemia, and hypoxia (Heegaard & Biros, 2007). These secondary injuries are related to poorer outcomes (Ghajar, 2000; Heegaard & Biros, 2007). Due to the complex pathophysiologic changes associated with TBI and the additional impact of secondary injury, clinical presentation is diverse.

Potential Impact on Communication/Swallowing

Cognitive-communication, language, speech, and swallowing impairments are common with TBI, especially those classified as moderate and severe. The most severe patients present with disorders of consciousness, referring to individuals who are in a coma, minimally conscious, or in a vegetative state. Approximately 80% of patients will recover consciousness (Dolce et al., 2015). As patients emerge, post-traumatic amnesia (PTA) is often present. The duration of PTA can be used as a prognostic indicator for overall recovery (Walker et al., 2010). PTA is generally longer in patients with diffuse brain injury than those with localized lesions (Levin, O'Donnell, & Grossman, 1979). The Orientation Log (Novack, 2000), Galveston Orientation and Amnesia Test (Levin et al., 1979) or Westmead PTA scale (Shores, Marosszeky, Sandanam, & Batchelor, 1986) are frequently used as assessments of PTA. Patients may present with confabulation (which is the belief that false memories are real), anterograde amnesia, and disorientation (Ponsford et al., 2004). Behavioral impairments may include aggression, agitation, and irritability, all of which will impact an individual's ability to attend to and participate in meaningful communication.

Even after the resolution of PTA, or in the case of patients who did not have PTA, a wide variety of cognitive-communication and social cognition (Allain et al., 2018) impairments are associated with TBI. Due to the variability of lesion site, as well as the impact of diffuse axonal injury, cerebral edema, and increased cranial pressure, patients can present with localized and/or diffuse impairments. Patients with TBI can manifest deficits in attention, retrospective and prospective memory, executive functions (such as planning and problem solving), and metacognition (Belmont, Agar, Hugeron, Gallais, & Azouvi, 2006; Kennedy & Coehlo, 2005; O'Brien & Kennedy, 2018). Narrative discourse deficits may be present after TBI, including decreased organization and completeness (Lindsey, Hurley, Mozeiko, & Coelho, 2018). Reduced processing speed is also common and has been linked to diffuse axonal injury (Felmingham, Baguley, & Green, 2004). Linguistic deficits can occur in patients with TBI, particularly those with left hemisphere lesions. Fatigue is also a common disability among people with TBI (Belmont et al., 2006) and may negatively impact cognitive-communication functioning.

Speech is disrupted in 10% to 60% of individuals with TBI (Mitchell, Bowen, Tyson, Butterfint, & Conroy, 2017). According to Duffy (2013), any type of dysarthria can occur secondary to a TBI, though spastic dysarthria is the most common for a closed head injury and flaccid dysarthria for a skull fracture. Aphonia may occur secondary to tracheostomy. According to Gurkin and colleagues (2002) the incidence of tracheostomy tube placement is 44% of patients with a GCS of <9.

Patients with TBI also frequently present with dysphagia. Risk factors for dysphagia associated with TBI include low Glasgow Coma Scale and Rancho Los Amigos scores, ventilation for 15 or more days, and CT scan revealing midline shift, brainstem involvement, or the need for emergent procedures (Mackay, Morgan, & Bernstein, 1999). Lee and colleagues (2016) compared dysphagic individuals with TBI to those with dysphagia secondary to stroke and found no significant difference in the severity or characteristics of dysphagia between the two groups; however, individuals with TBI who had surgical intervention, such as craniectomy or craniotomy, were at increased risk for tube feedings. The impairments seen most frequently in both groups were aspiration or penetration, decreased laryngeal elevation, and reduced epiglottic inversion (Lee et al., 2016). Oral phase deficits may also be present in patients with TBI, exacerbated by attentional deficits and reduced self-monitoring. Cognitive skills play a role in the safety of patients with TBI during meals.

Role of the SLP

The SLP is an integral member of the rehabilitation team for patients with acquired brain injury. In the acute care setting, initial assessment may be limited to dysphagia and awareness/orientation. Cognitive-communication and language screenings may be completed; however, achieving medical stability will be the primary goal of the patient's care team. The hospital SLP should closely monitor the patient, including via frequent chart review. Feeling comfortable reading reports from neurology and radiology (e.g., brain CT and MRI) is important.

Although there is substantial overlap in the assessment and treatment of speech, swallowing, cognitive-communication, and language, there are a few specific considerations for TBI. For example, it will be important to note the patient's level on the Rancho Los Amigos Scale. This can generally be found in a physician's note and will provide valuable guidance to the evaluating clinician (Table 2–1). For example, a patient who is reported to be a Rancho Level II (generalized responses) will only be appropriate for an assessment of responsiveness rather than a standardized test of language. Early treatment with patients at these low levels (Rancho Levels I to III) generally includes sensory stimulation through tactile, olfactory, auditory, and taste input (Dolce and colleagues, 2015; Pape and colleagues, 2015). By comparison, a patient at Rancho Level VI is emerging from post-traumatic amnesia and may attend to highly familiar tasks for a short period and learn to use a memory book with maximum assistance.

For patients with TBI and stroke, dysphagia assessment will be an early priority for the hospital SLP. Clinical assessment can provide useful information regarding a patient's overall status which may impact ability to participate in formal assessment and/or oral intake. This includes alertness/arousal, respiratory status, cognitive-communication skills, and behavior. Depending on the individual's presentation, food and liquid trials may be presented as an initial assessment, a recommendation may be made for an instrumental study (e.g., VFSS, FEES), or it may be necessary to closely monitor until the person is more appropriate. Diet modification may be warranted, as well as feeding supervision and compensatory strategies. A growing body of literature exists to support dysphagia rehabilitation, incorporating many principles of motor learning and neuroplasticity (Crary Carnaby, LaGorio, & Carvajal, 2012; Malandraki et al., 2016; Morgan, 2017; Rangarathnam & McCullough, 2017; Robbins et al., 2007). Exercise-based treatment likely will not occur until the

Table 2–1. Summary of Rancho Los Amigos Levels of Cognitive Functioning

Rancho Level	Description	Assessment	Treatment
Level I	No response	DOCS[a], JFK-CRS[b]	Sensory stimulation
Level II	Generalized response		
Level III	Localized response		
Level IV	Confused, agitated	Orientation assessment, Dysphagia assessment	Dysphagia treatment/management, Orientation, Awareness
Level V	Confused, inappropriate		
Level VI	Confused, appropriate	Orientation assessment, Dysphagia assessment, Possibly formal assessment of cognition/language	Dysphagia treatment/management, Orientation, Awareness, +other appropriate cognitive-communication or language goal areas
Level VII	Automatic, appropriate	Any appropriate formal assessment	All appropriate goal areas
Level VIII	Purposeful, appropriate		

Notes. [a]Disorders of Consciousness Scale (Pape, Heinemann, Kelly, Hurder, & Lundgren, 2005). [b]JFK Coma Recovery Scale-Revised (Giacino, Kalmar, & Whyte, 2004).

patient has transferred to a rehabilitation setting; however, exercises should be considered early, especially in the case of patients who are unable to eat or drink by mouth.

Assessing and facilitating basic communication is important in the acute care setting. Individuals with tracheostomies may benefit from an alternate form of communication, such as writing or pictures, or placement of a speaking valve (Batty, 2009). An individual with dysarthria may benefit from postural adjustments or training in compensatory strategies, such as slowing rate or modifying the speech-breathing pattern (Spencer & Brown., 2018). Alphabet or pacing boards may be beneficial (Yorkston et al., 2010). Use of AAC, such as picture boards, is often effective for patients with aphasia in the controlled hospital environment (Jacobs, Drew, Ogletree, & Pierce, 2004). Family and staff education will be especially important, ensuring that they understand how to set the environment, interact with the patient, and facilitate effective communication.

Direct intervention for impairment level deficits, such as language, memory, and attention, will likely be limited in an acute care setting; however, it is important to be aware of evidence-based methods that may be implemented once the patient is more stable. For example, there is a wealth of literature supporting aphasia treatment, which can be applied to individuals with stroke and TBI. These include methods such as Oral Reading for Language in Aphasia (ORLA; Cherney, 2010), Constraint-Induced Language Therapy (CILT; Pulvermüller et al., 2001), Semantic Feature Analysis (SFA; Efstratiadou, Papathanasiou, Holland, Archonti, & Hilari, 2018), and Verb Network Strengthening Treatment (VneST; Edmonds, 2016), to name a few. Melodic Intonation Therapy (MIT; Sparks, Helm, & Albert, 1974) is sometimes used with patients presenting with co-occurring aphasia and apraxia of speech, though more recent, evidence-based approaches would include treatments such as Sound Production Treatment (SPT; Wambaugh, Wright, & Mauszycki, 2014, 2013). There is positive evidence for interventions targeting many aspects of cognition, including memory, attention, social communication, visuospatial deficits, and executive functions, in patients with TBI and stroke (Cicerone et al., 2011). Training metacognitive strategies is especially important for those with TBI.

NEURODEGENERATIVE DISORDERS

Rene Ruzicka Kanadet

Neurodegenerative diseases are caused by deterioration of neurons in the brain and/or spinal cord. The rate of these diagnoses is expected to increase over the next several decades due to the aging population and increased lifespan (NIH, 2018). At this time, according to the Harvard NeuroDiscovery Center, five million Americans are diagnosed with Alzheimer's disease; one million with Parkinson's disease; 400,000 with multiple sclerosis (MS); 30,000 with amyotrophic lateral sclerosis (ALS, or Lou Gehrig's disease); and 30,000 with Huntington's disease (accessed 2018). While this list is not exhaustive, it captures many of the diagnoses commonly seen by the hospital SLP.

Dementia

Description of the Medical Condition

Dementia is a condition marked by a functional decline in cognitive and/or behavioral symptoms not related to a delirium or major psychiatric disorder (McKhann et al., 2011).

Impairments may include the inability to learn and recall new information; impaired reasoning and judgment; decreased visuospatial abilities, such as difficulty recognizing faces or common objects; impaired language skills; and changes in personality or behavior, such as agitation, social withdrawal, or compulsive behaviors (McKhann et al., 2011). Types of dementia include Alzheimer's dementia, Lewy body dementia, fronto-temporal dementia, and vascular dementia (Smits et al., 2015). The *Diagnostic and Statistical Manual of Mental Disorders* (5th ed.; *DSM–5*; American Psychiatric Association, 2013) now refers to dementia as "major neurocognitive disorder," though the terms continue to be used interchangeably.

Potential Impact on Communication/Swallowing

As described above, cognitive changes are the primary symptoms of dementia, however language impairments increase as the disease progresses. Word finding difficulties are primary in the early stages of dementia, with more noticeable impairments in middle/late stages, characterized by semantic emptiness, and at times becoming nonverbal (Watson, Aizawa, Savundranayagam, & Orange, 2013). Language comprehension also decreases with disease progression. Communication is further impacted negatively by reduced attention, memory, recognition, and behavioral changes. These cognitive-communication impairments negatively affect a person's activities of daily living and, ultimately, their ability to live independently.

Patients with dementia are at increased risk for aspiration. Dysphagia is present in later stage dementia, with diffuse brain lesions impacting the sensorimotor aspects of the swallowing sequence (Rogus-Pulia, Malandraki, Johnson, & Robbins, 2015). Safety during eating is significantly impacted by cognitive impairments in dementia. For example, patients may demonstrate decreased ability to identify, recall, and utilize appropriate utensils during eating; poor attention during mealtimes; decreased ability to self-feed; impulsivity; apathy during meals; and reduced ability to follow instructions. It is suggested that these cognitive impairments may cause difficulty with eating in the early stages of dementia, even before sensorimotor aspects of swallowing have been impacted (Rogus-Pulia et al., 2015). Patients with dementia may also hold/pocket food in their mouths for extended periods of time. Rogus-Pulia and colleagues (2015) summarized swallow study (VFSS and FEES) findings for individuals with dementia, including: longer oral transit times, reduced pharyngeal clearance, and penetration/aspiration in *Alzheimer's disease*; reduced bolus formation and mastication, decreased hyolaryngeal movement, and reduced epiglottic inversion in *vascular dementia*; delayed pharyngeal initiation, pharyngeal residue, and penetration/aspiration in *Lewy body dementia*; and rapid, compulsive eating, large bolus volumes, premature spillage into the pharynx, and pharyngeal residue in *fronto-temporal dementia*. Poor oral care in those with dementia is an additional contributor to aspiration pneumonia risk.

Parkinson's Disease

Description of Medical Condition

Parkinson's disease (PD) is a progressive movement disorder. It is characterized by tremor at rest, rigidity, bradykinesia, postural instability, flexed posture, and freezing (Jankovic, 2008). Additional nonmotor symptoms often include changes in sleep, smell, and cognition. Age of onset is generally between 55 and 75 years. Severity of symptoms may be rated by the Hoehn and Yahr Scale (Goetz et al., 2007; Hoehn & Yahr, 1967), which ranges from stage 0 (no signs of disease) to 5 (wheelchair bound or bedridden unless assisted), or the Unified Parkinson's Disease Rating Scale (UPDRS; Goetz et al., 2007), a comprehensive rating system used to track the motor and nonmotor characteristics of PD. Motor symptoms are attributed to degeneration of dopamine-producing neurons within the substantia nigra pars compacta. Presence of a-synuclein, a substance in Lewy bodies, is also indicated in PD (Exner, Lutz, Haass, & Winklhofer, 2012). PD is treated with dopamine-replacement medications, such as Levodopa, to reduce severity of symptoms. Deep brain stimulation (DBS) to the globus pallidus or subthalamic nucleus is also used, either in combination with Levodopa or in an effort to reduce drug therapy due to intolerance (St. George, Nutt, Burchiel, & Horiak, 2010).

Potential Impact on Communication/Swallowing

Hypokinetic dysarthria is typically associated with PD. Distinctive characteristics include reduced vocal intensity, monopitch, mono-loudness, decreased articulatory precision, and accelerated rushes of speech (Duffy, 2013). Palilalia, or compulsive repetition of words or phrases, may also occur in patients with PD. Cognitive-communication impairments are common, with cognitive deficits ranging from mild cognitive impairment (MCI) to dementia (Litvan et al., 2012). Early cognitive impairments are reported in executive function, attention, visuospatial skills, and memory, notably retrieval skills (Nazem et al., 2009). Mild cognitive impairment is reportedly present in anywhere from 35% to 42.5% of patients at the time of diagnosis, and 50% will be diagnosed with dementia within 10 years (Cosgrove, Alty, & Jamieson, 2015).

Dysphagia is a common condition associated with PD, occurring in approximately 80% of individuals with PD (Kalf, de Swart, Bloem, & Munnecke, 2012). Reported oral phase deficits include reduced bolus formation and mastication, delayed initiation, tongue pumping, premature spillage into the pharynx, piecemeal deglutition, and oral residue. Pharyngeal phase deficits include delayed laryngeal movement, reduced epiglottic inversion, and decreased pharyngeal constriction, resulting in pharyngeal residue and increased rates of penetration and aspiration (Michou, Baijens, Rofes, Cartgena, & Clave, 2013). Lingual weakness may also be implicated in dysphagia (Pitts, Morales, & Stierwalt, 2018).

Multiple Sclerosis

Description of Medical Condition

Multiple sclerosis (MS) is a chronic, inflammatory, autoimmune disease of the central nervous system and is cited as one of the most common causes of neurological disability in young adults (NIH, 2018). The initial symptoms of MS typically occur between 20 and 50 years of age, and women are approximately 3 times more likely to develop MS compared with men (Gooch, Pracht, & Borenstein, 2017). Interestingly, the prevalence of MS varies by geographic location, and generally increases the further one travels from the equator (Simpson, Blizzard, Otahal, Van der Mei, & Taylor, 2011). Reasons for this geographic influence are not entirely clear, but may be linked to vitamin D deficiency or genetic differences.

Multiple sclerosis is marked by damage to the myelin sheath of neurons in the brain and spinal cord with clinical manifestations dependent upon what neurons have been affected. These may include changes in movement, sensory perception, cognitive function, speech, and swallowing. Differential diagnosis is often difficult with MS due to similar presentation with diseases including Lyme disease, lupus, and paraneoplastic disease (McDonald et al., 2001). There are four types of MS with relapse-remitting being the most common. This type of MS is characterized by exacerbation periods followed by recovery/remission, though full recovery between relapses may not occur, and progressive decline is seen over time. Additional types of MS include primary-progressive, characterized by progressive deterioration from onset; secondary-progressive, with initial relapsing-remitting followed by progression; and progressive-relapsing multiple sclerosis, characterized by acute relapses but with continuing progression between relapses (Miller & Leary, 2007).

Potential Impact on Communication/Swallowing

Dysphagia, dysarthria, and cognitive-communication impairments are possible in patients with MS. The clinical presentation is dependent upon what areas of the brain have been affected by demyelination and neurodegeneration. Dysarthria can be any type, with spastic-ataxic being the most commonly cited mixed dysarthria (Duffy, 2013). Speech characteristics associated with MS include reduced volume control; harsh voice; imprecise articulation; impaired stress patterns, rate, and breath support; and variable pitch (Darley, Brown, & Goldstein, 1972; Hartelius, Theodoros, Cahill, & Lillvik, 2003).

Cognitive changes may occur early, preceding physical impairments, and can occur with any type of MS (Patti, 2009), though it is highest in the secondary progressive population (Trenova et al., 2016). Presentation is heterogeneous, though impairments are most commonly seen in memory, attention, processing speed, visuospatial skills, and executive functions. Fatigue and depression may also contribute to cognitive-communication deficits (Patti, 2009; Trenova et al., 2016).

Dysphagia is reported in anywhere from 17% to 65% of patients with MS (Giusti & Giambuzzi, 2008; Tassorelli et al., 2008). Characteristics of dysphagia include impairments in the oral phase due to lingual, labial, and/or velar involvement; premature spillage of material into the pharynx and/or larynx; impaired tongue base retraction; decreased pharyngeal contraction; reduced laryngeal closure; and decreased pharyngeal and/or laryngeal sensation (Prosiegel, Schelling, & Wagner-Sonntag, 2004; Tassorelli et al., 2008). These impairments result in decreased oral and pharyngeal clearance, penetration/aspiration, and apnea during or after eating (Giusti & Giambuzzi, 2008; Tassorelli et al., 2008). Some patients with MS also have decreased relaxation of the upper esophageal sphincter, which contributes to pharyngeal residue (Giusti & Giambuzzi, 2008; Prosiegel, Schelling, & Wagner-Sonntag, 2004; Tassorelli et al., 2008).

Amyotrophic Lateral Sclerosis

Description of Medical Condition

Amyotrophic lateral sclerosis (ALS) is a mixed upper and lower motor neuron disease characterized by degeneration of motor neurons in the brain and spinal cord. Typical age of onset is mid-to-late 50s, and death usually occurs within 3 to 5 years (Brown & AlChalabi, 2017). Most cases of ALS begin with limb weakness, eventually spreading to most muscles, including those of respiration. Approximately one-third of cases, however, are bulbar, which is characterized by earlier difficulty speaking and swallowing. Pseudobulbar affect may be seen. Some patients with ALS will also present with fronto-temporal dementia. Additional types of motor neuron disease include progressive muscle atrophy (PMA), primary lateral sclerosis, and progressive bulbar palsy

(PBP), though ALS represents approximately 80% of total cases (Chieia, Oliveira, Silva, & Gabbai, 2010).

Potential Impact on Communication/Swallowing

Dysarthria and dysphagia occur in all patients with ALS, though persons with bulbar onset will experience severe speech and swallowing symptoms earlier in the disease progression. The typical dysarthria associated with ALS is mixed spastic-flaccid due to involvement of the upper and lower motor neurons (Duffy, 2013). This dysarthria commonly manifests as slow rate of speech, imprecise articulation, hypernasality, monopitch, and harsh or breathy vocal quality. As the disease progresses, 80% to 95% of people with ALS will become unable to use natural speech for functional communication, and most will lose their ability to speak (Beukelman, Fager, & Nordness, 2011).

Dysphagia is one of the earliest symptoms in individuals with ALS with a bulbar onset, though it occurs in all patients with ALS and typically leads to percutaneous endoscopic gastrostomy (PEG) placement for enteral nutrition. Dysphagia symptoms include chewing fatigue, drooling, nasopharyngeal reflux, coughing and choking, impaired bolus formation, and difficulty with oral transit (Hadjikoutis & Wiles, 2001). Early dysphagia in ALS patients was described by Teissman et al. (2011) as primarily pharyngeal, characterized by weak pharyngeal constriction and residue in the valleculae and pyriforms, whereas impaired bolus preparation and transit was evident in more severely impaired patients. Atypical respiratory patterns are also present during swallowing with inspiration after the swallow, longer apnea during the swallow, and multiple swallows per bolus (Hadjikoutis & Wiles, 2001).

Cognitive deficits are evident in approximately 30% of patients with ALS and are characterized by impairments in fluency, language, social cognition, verbal memory, and executive functions (Beeldman et al., 2016). It is estimated that 15% to 20% of ALS patients will present with fronto-temporal dementia (Abrahams, Newton, Niven, Foley, & Bak, 2014; Brown & Al-Chalabi, 2017); the co-occurrence of these disorders has been linked to genetic mutations (Turner et al., 2017). Frontotemporal dementia (FTD) is marked by behavioral and personality changes.

Huntington's Disease

Description of Medical Condition

Huntington's disease (HD) is an autosomal-dominant genetic disorder. The primary motor characteristic is chorea, which is characterized by involuntary jerking and writhing movements. Other common symptoms include dystonia, incoordination, slow saccadic eye movement, cognitive decline, motor impersistence, and behavioral changes (O'Walker, 2007). The age of onset for HD is typically middle-age though a juvenile onset is possible between the ages of 2 and 20. Genetic testing can be completed to confirm HD even before symptoms present. Although there is no treatment to slow disease progression, management strategies may include pharmacological treatment of chorea and pharmacological and nonpharmacological treatment of psychiatric and behavioral disturbances (Frank, 2014).

Potential Impact on Communication/Swallowing

Cognitive impairments are a hallmark characteristic of HD and impact participation in daily living tasks and communication situations.

Impairments are seen in attention; memory; visuospatial processing; executive functions, including problem solving, thought flexibility, and planning; and emotional processing, including interpretation of emotions through facial expression and voice (Montoya, Price, Menear, & Lepage, 2006). These deficits become severe in later stages of the disease.

Speech intelligibility is impacted by choreic movements, resulting in a hyperkinetic dysarthria. The severity of the person's dysarthria is related to the severity of the chorea. Movements of the jaw, tongue, and lips can affect articulation. Irregular articulatory breakdowns, prolonged phonemes, and abnormal lengthening of vowels are characteristic (Duffy, 2013). Unpredictable movements can also result in changes in respiration, such as forced and involuntary inspiration or expiration; volume, such as excess loudness; and vocal quality, including a strained vocal quality or voice arrest.

Dysphagia is likely to occur as HD progresses (O'Walker, 2007). Characteristics of dysphagia with chorea include rapid lingual movements, decreased coordination of the swallow, prolonged laryngeal elevation, and poor coordination of respiration and swallowing (Kagel & Leopold, 1992). Kagel and Leopold (1992) further described that bradykinesia in patients with HD can lead to mandibular rigidity, slow lingual chorea, and coughing on foods and liquids. Pharyngeal retention and aspiration were identified through videofluoroscopy in this same study. Self-feeding is also an issue for patients with HD (Bilney, Morris, & Perry, 2003). Involuntary movements may limit the ability to bring food and utensils to the mouth in a controlled manner, causing reduced oral acceptance and control and/or anterior loss. Body movements may also increase aspiration risk. In a retrospective study by Heemskirk and Roos (2012), 55% of the reviewed patients died of pneumonia, and a majority of these patients could be further identified as having aspiration pneumonia.

Role of the SLP in Neurodegenerative Disorders

The role of the SLP changes with disease progression and may start before there has even been a confirmed diagnosis. A thorough oral mechanism exam and evaluation of speech and swallowing may offer neurologists and other medical providers valuable information during the diagnostic process. These evaluations, in addition to assessment of cognitive-communication, should be completed at all phases of disease progression.

At early stages of disease, an important role of the SLP is education, especially when there are no overt symptoms of dysphagia, dysarthria, or cognitive-communication deficits. It is known that most persons with neurodegenerative diagnoses will experience these impairments, as described above; therefore, it is important to consider educating the patient and family on what to expect, when to seek medical attention, and the role of the SLP throughout the progression of their disease. Education on clinical signs of aspiration and other warning signs for dysphagia, such as weight loss, fevers, and pneumonia is especially important. It is also important that the SLP complete assessments in these early stages. Subtle signs of dysphagia, dysarthria, and cognitive-communication changes may not be reported. Underreporting of symptoms may occur secondary to progressive adaptation to slow changes. Assessments are warranted to identify impairments and encourage early intervention and/or to serve as a baseline for future assessments.

Continued assessment is important at all phases of disease progression in order to provide updated recommendations, especially with regards to dysphagia, as aspiration pneumonia is a leading cause of death in these populations (Walshe, 2014). Patients with previous knowledge of their dysphagia may be resistant to further diagnostics or feel that they are already well informed. Provide education and encouragement. Diet modifications and compensatory strategy training are important as neurodegeneration progresses. Cognitive abilities should always be taken into consideration when making recommendations, and family or caregiver training is crucial.

When the progression of the disease has become very severe, advanced diagnostics, such as VFSS, may not be appropriate. A discussion with the patient's family to determine priorities and end-of-life wishes should occur prior to completing these tests. Quality of life must always be considered. It is imperative that the SLP provide thorough education on dysphagia and the risks of an unrestricted diet; however, the patient/family's decision must always be respected. Including the patient's physician on the conversation is recommended when discussing diet liberalization.

During an acute hospitalization, patients with neurodegenerative diseases will likely be encountered with a different admitting diagnosis. For example, a patient with dementia may be admitted for pneumonia, or a patient with PD may be admitted following a fall and subsequent hip fracture. In these cases, the SLP may not be consulted or may be consulted for an isolated assessment, such as swallowing. During short admissions, or when a patient is acutely ill, treatment of speech, swallowing, and/or cognitive-communication skills may not be feasible or a priority; however, referral to rehabilitation services should be encouraged. Initial education to patients and families on the rationale for intervention may increase understanding and follow-through post-discharge from the acute care setting. SLP recommendations may also contribute to physician decision making regarding next level of care, for example, if considering discharge home or to inpatient rehabilitation.

Although not curative, there is positive evidence for rehabilitation with neurodegenerative populations. Lee Silverman Voice Treatment (LSVT) is a well-known example of treatment for patients with dysarthria related to PD (Sapir, Spielman, Ramig, Story, & Fox, 2007). Use of expiratory muscle strength training (EMST) has shown improvements in maximum expiratory pressure and hyolaryngeal elevation in ALS (Plowman et al., 2016) and PD (Troche et al., 2010), as well as improving cough strength in patients with moderate MS (Chiara, Martin, Davenport, & Bolser, 2006). Cognitive-communication treatment may include strategy training and use of repeated cognitive exercises resulting in a training effect (Lovera & Kovner, 2012). Spaced Retrieval Training (SRT) has shown success in increasing new learning in patients with dementia (Hopper et al., 2013; Oren, Willerton, & Small, 2014), as well as use of SRT paired with external aids for compliance with swallow strategies (Benigas & Bourgeois, 2016). Alternative and augmentative communication (AAC) should be considered as a supplement or alternative to verbal communication for patients with dysarthria. This may be low-tech, such as use of an alphabet board or writing, or a high-tech speech generating device (Fried-Oken, Mooney, & Peters, 2015). Numerous access methods for speech generating devices are available for individuals with pronounced physical limitations, such as eye gaze, head movement, or foot movement. Providing and training use of an AAC device is recommended early in the progression of diseases, such as ALS, and is associated with increased quality of life (Körner et al., 2013).

Specific diagnosis, stage of progression, previous SLP assessment and treatment, and patient/family wishes must all be considered when a patient with a neurodegenerative diagnosis is encountered. Speech, swallowing, and cognitive-communication skills should be evaluated in patients with these diagnoses, regardless of reported symptoms. The hospital SLP has an important role in education and evaluation, as well as rehabilitation, in these settings.

ENCEPHALOPATHY

Rene Ruzicka Kanadet

Encephalopathy refers to any diffuse disease of the brain that causes a clinical state of altered mental status. Manifestations include disorientation, confusion, behavioral changes, and other cognitive impairments (Venkatesan et al., 2013). There are several causes of encephalopathy, including metabolic dysfunction, exposure to toxins, hypoxia/anoxia, chronic progressive trauma, and bacterial or viral infectious agents (National Institute of Neurological Disorders and Stroke, 2018a).

Toxic-Metabolic Encephalopathies

Toxic-metabolic encephalopathies are due to an underlying disorder and lead to diffuse neurological symptoms. Toxic encephalopathy is caused by alcohol, drug, or chemical toxicity (National Institute of Neurological Disorders and Stroke, 2018b). Causes of metabolic encephalopathies include metabolic disorders, vitamin deficiency, and organ failure. Both toxic and metabolic encephalopathies present with global, nonfocal deficits, such as confusion, delirium, or hallucinations, with a widespread pattern of brain injury involving the deep gray nuclei and cerebral cortex (Kim & Kim, 2012; Sharma, Eesa, & Scott, 2009). Presentation can be acute or chronic.

Acute toxic-metabolic encephalopathy is characterized by a rapid onset of altered mental status. Sepsis is the most frequent cause of encephalopathy in ICU settings (Ziaja, 2013). The cause of sepsis-associated encephalopathy is complex, with inflammatory and noninflammatory processes affecting brain cells with specific breakdown of the blood-brain barrier (Iacobone et al., 2009; Ziaja, 2013). It has also been described as a metabolic encephalopathy (Zauner et al., 2000). An example of vitamin deficiency-related encephalopathy is Wernicke's encephalopathy, which is caused by thiamine deficiency (Flynn, Macaluso, D'Empaire, & Troutman, 2015). Heroin and cocaine are among the recreational drugs known for causing encephalopathy (Valk & van der Knaap, 1992; Sharma et al., 2009). Pharmaceuticals including cyclosporine and ifomosfamide are also indicated (Sharma et al., 2009; Hamadani & Awan, 2006). Solvents, gasses, and heavy metals can cause neurotoxicity (Kim & Kim, 2012). Cognitive dysfunction including impairments in consciousness; it generally including coma, are prominent, as well as seizures. Delirium is commonly cited in acute toxic and metabolic encephalopathies; it generally resolves when the underlying disorder is treated or the toxic element is eliminated from the body.

Chronic toxic-metabolic encephalopathy may go undetected for many years, but is known to be caused by organ failure, chronic alcohol abuse, and chronic exposure to toxins. Minimal hepatic encephalopathy (HE) in individuals with liver dysfunction, for example, is characterized by cognitive changes detectable on testing even when overt symptoms are not noted (Bajaj, 2010). Minimal HE is often undetected without specific testing due to preserved general mental status (Bajaj, 2010) and verbal abilities (Weissenborn, Ennen, Schomerus, Rueckert, & Hecker, 2001). These patients perform more poorly on tests of psychomotor speed, visual perception and attention, working memory, and executive functions (Bajaj, 2010; Weissenborn et al., 2001). Safety while driving and participation in activities of daily living can be impacted. Diabetic encephalopathy can emerge as a result of Type1 diabetes secondary to white matter atrophy in the frontal and temporal regions, as well as structural gray matter deficits in limbic structures (Sima et al., 2009). Like hepatic encephalopathy, cognitive deficits are noted in memory, executive functions, attention, and processing speed. In the case of chronic exposure to toxins, including chronic drug or alcohol abuse or environmental exposure to chemicals, permanent damage can occur with slow changes to cognitive and motor skills over time.

Chronic Traumatic Encephalopathy

Chronic traumatic encephalopathy (CTE) occurs when an individual has experienced repetitive brain trauma, such as from sports. CTE is a tau pathology, or tauopathy, which stems from a pathological clustering of tau protein in the brain. It is characterized by abnormal tau, distributed in an irregular pattern, in neurons and astroglia in small blood vessels at the depths of cortical sulci (McKee, Cairns, Dickson, Folkerth et al., 2016). Additional, supportive, but non-specific pathological features of CTE include pretangles of tau affecting superficial layers of cerebral cortex and the hippocampus, as well as neuronal and astrocytic clusters of tau in subcortical nuclei (McKee et al., 2016). At present, CTE cannot be definitely diagnosed until autopsy.

Chronic traumatic encephalopathy shares similarities with many neurodegenerative disorders. Previous reports of the CTE clinical syndrome include broad, nonspecific impairment in cognitive functioning (e.g., memory, executive function, and processing

speed), behavior (e.g., aggression, paranoia, and impulsivity), and mood (e.g., depression, anxiety, and suicidality), though researchers have questioned the existence of such a characteristic profile (see Asken, Sullan, DeKosky, Jaffee, & Bauer, 2017; McKee et al., 2009).

Encephalitis

It is important to differentiate the term encephalitis from encephalopathy. These labels are frequently used in similar contexts; however, delineation helps to ensure appropriate treatment (Chaudhuri & Kennedy, 2002). Whereas encephalopathy refers to any diffuse disease of the brain that causes a clinical state of altered mental status, encephalitis occurs when there is inflammation of the brain parenchyma, most commonly caused by a viral infection. Herpes simplex virus, West Nile virus, and varicella zoster virus are frequently cited as viral causes (Venkatesan, 2015; Venkatesan et al., 2013), though over 100 infectious causes have been reported (Thakur et al., 2013). A recent review describing the advances in epidemiology of acute encephalitis notes a growing number of autoimmune diseases that are also linked to this brain inflammation (Venkatesan, 2015). Thakur et al. (2013) reviewed a sample of individuals with encephalitis who received ICU care and noted poorer outcomes in those with autoimmune causes. Medical management is complex, especially given the challenge of differential diagnosis. Neurological symptoms may be generalized or focal, and seizures are common (Venkatesan, 2015; Chaudhuri & Kennedy, 2002). In some, encephalitis can present as flu-like symptoms, such as headache, fever, fatigue, and muscle aches. However, in others, the symptoms are more severe, such as confusion, agitation, muscle weakness, seizures, speech difficulty, or loss of consciousness. Coma can occur in severe cases (Chaudhuri & Kennedy, 2002). Patients may be treated with antivirals, anticonvulsants, and steroids while hospitalized.

HIV-Related Encephalitis and Encephalopathy

Human immunodeficiency virus (HIV) can cause both encephalopathy and encephalitis. Tauber et al. (2016) describe a continuum of neuroinflammation, causing a range of impairment, from mild neurocognitive disorders to HIV-encephalitis, also known as HIV or AIDS dementia. Individuals with AIDS dementia will demonstrate a gradual decline in cognitive and motor function. Characteristics of HIV encephalopathy include widening of ventricles, brain atrophy, neuronal loss in the hippocampal formation, and perivascular demyelination (Tauber et al., 2016). It should be noted that individuals with HIV/AIDS are also at increased risk for opportunistic infections, which could cause encephalitis, such as cytomegalovirus, herpes, and toxoplasma (National Institute of Neurological Disorders and Stroke, 2018c).

Potential Impact on Communication/Swallowing

Brain damage associated with encephalopathy and encephalitis is often diffuse, though encephalitis can also result in localized damage. For example, Tyler (2004) reported aphasia as a symptom at the time of hospital admission in 76% of the study population. Symptoms may be mild or severe and are related to the areas of involvement in the brain.

Cognitive impairments predominate. Altered consciousness, including coma, is common in both encephalopathy and encephalitis (Venkatesan, 2015). Disorientation and confusion may be present, as well as cognitive changes including reduced attention, memory,

and executive functions (Bajaj, 2010; Tyler, 2004). Cognitive changes may persist after resolution of acute symptoms (Ziaja, 2013).

Dysphagia and dysarthria may be present, depending upon the areas of the brain that are impacted. For example, dysphagia and dysarthria are reported as a symptom in patients with brainstem encephalitis (Deitrich-Burns, Lewis, Lesley, & Solomon, 2013). Prolonged intubation may cause or exacerbate a dysphagia. Cognitive impairments may decrease safety during meals, thus increasing aspiration risk or putting the individual at nutritional risk.

Chronic traumatic encephalopathy differs from encephalitis and other types of encephalopathy due to the neurodegenerative nature. McKee and colleagues (2009) reported movement symptoms in 41% of the study population, including dysarthria and dysphagia. As previously discussed, the cognitive-communication changes include memory loss, reduced attention, and disorientation. Communication skills are further impacted by changes in personality and behavior, which can impact interpersonal relationships. Disease progression often includes Parkinsonism and dementia; therefore, clinical manifestations related to speech, cognitive-communications skills, and swallowing associated with these diagnoses should be expected.

Role of the SLP

The hospital SLP is likely to encounter patients with encephalopathy and encephalitis across levels of care, with a notable concentration in ICU settings. Early during admissions, the SLP may be consulted to evaluate swallowing in the setting of altered mental status, delirium, or confusion. Without a confirmed encephalopathy or encephalitis diagnosis, these clinical descriptors should be considered red flags. Safest diet and supervision recommendations should be made, and the SLP should continue with close monitoring for several days, as status may be changing rapidly.

SLPs should consider if the patient had been intubated and for how long, as the prevalence of postextubation dysphagia ranges from 44% to 87% (Ajemian, Nirmul, Anderson, Zirlen, & Kwasnik, 2001; Moraes, Sassi, Mangilli, Zilberstein, & de Andrade, 2013). Generalized weakness is an additional consideration, as many patients with encephalopathy have weakness from chronic illness or may have been receiving enteral nutrition for a period of time while acutely ill, intubated, and/or sedated. Instrumental tests of swallowing (VFSS and FEES) should be completed throughout the hospitalization to ensure the safest diet. Fiberendoscopic evaluation of swallowing (FEES) has added clinical utility in the ICU, as several examinations may be warranted in a short period of time due to status changes, and there is no radiation exposure. FEES can also be completed at bedside. Mental status should guide recommendations for swallow safety.

Monitoring mental status will also be an early goal of the SLP, including assessment of arousal, alertness, and orientation. In cases of acute encephalopathy and encephalitis, there is an expectation of improvement in symptoms when the underlying disease has been treated. Close communication with the medical team and review of the medical chart will be important, to determine the best time to complete further dysarthria and cognitive-communication testing. Treatment is appropriate when the patient is medically stable, no longer in a state of delirium, sedated, and/or in active drug or alcohol withdrawal. Cognitive-communication or language testing should be completed with patients under SLP care, even when it is believed that symptoms have fully resolved, as evidence suggests high rates of persistent cognitive deficits. Individuals recovering from encephalitis will require

rehabilitation of cognitive-communication skills, swallowing, and speech. Treatment recommendations will vary based on clinical presentation.

The hospital SLP should also consider assessment of patients with chronic diseases, such as liver disease, diabetes, COPD, and history of drug or alcohol abuse. Although these patients may not present with an acute encephalopathy, it is known that there are often cognitive changes over time. Completing testing or making a referral to neuropsychology is appropriate. Treatment may include compensatory strategy training or cognitive rehabilitation. This also applies to CTE, which may not present with acute changes but warrants assessment. CTE should be treated as a neurodegenerative disorder.

PSYCHIATRIC DISORDERS

Doreen Kelly Izaguirre with Kristie A. Spencer

Psychiatric disorders in both adults and children will likely be encountered by the speech-language pathologist working in the medical setting, given the potential impact on communication, speech, and swallowing. Coverage of the full spectrum of psychiatric disorders is beyond the scope of this chapter; numerous general resources are available, including information from the American Psychiatric Association (APA). Speech-language pathology service delivery nicely complements the International Classification of Functioning, Disability, and Health (ICF) from the World Health Organization (WHO), especially when supporting individuals with psychiatric challenges. Psychiatric disturbances and conditions can often cloud the diagnostic profile for the speech-language pathologist. Referrals for both evaluation and treatment might include any combination of disorders, including cognitive-communication, language, motor speech, and swallowing.

The speech-language pathologist must be aware of the many psychiatric conditions and sequelae that may complicate the overall presentation of the patient. Knowledge of medications and the interventions used to address different psychiatric conditions is essential. Antipsychotic medications, otherwise known as neuroleptics, can potentially impact speech, swallowing, and cognition, with both short- and long-term effects. For example, recent research suggests that higher lifetime antipsychotic dose may be associated with poorer cognitive functioning (Husa et al., 2017). Psychiatric medications have also been described as a trade-off between alleviating symptoms of the psychiatric disorder and managing the results of the potential extrapyramidal symptoms, including tardive dyskinesia and dystonia, as well as the anticholinergic effects that include cognitive impairment (Muench & Hamer, 2010). Additionally, neuroleptic medications can also lead to dysphagia (Aldridge & Taylor, 2012; see Chapter 3 of this book for more information). Although there are numerous psychiatric disturbances that may impact cognitive-communication skills and swallowing that the speech-language pathologist may encounter in the medical setting, attention-deficit/hyperactivity disorder (ADHD), schizophrenia/schizoaffective disorders, and delirium are discussed here.

Attention-Deficit/Hyperactivity Disorder (ADHD)

Nature of ADHD

As noted by the American Psychiatric Association (APA, 2018), attention-deficit/hyperactivity disorder is one of the most prevalent mental health disorders impacting children and can also be seen in adults. ADHD is estimated to occur in 8.4% of children and 2.5% of adults (APA, 2018). There is some controversy over whether attention-deficit/hyperactivity disorder falls into the category of psychiatric disorders, yet simply, it involves mental functioning and can cause significant disruption to daily functioning. The *Diagnostic and Statistical Manual of Mental Disorders* (5th ed.; *DSM-5* American Psychiatric Association [APA], 2013) distinguishes three subtypes of ADHD: the predominantly inattentive type, the predominantly hyperactive/impulsive type, and the combined type. ADHD of the inattentive type leads to problems with attention and concentration, distractibility, organization skills, and task completion (APA, 2013; Paul, 2012). The hyperactivity/impulsive type may involve fidgeting, difficulty staying seated, acting without thinking, and talking too much (APA, 2013; Paul, 2013).

Patients with attention-deficit/hyperactivity disorder in the medical setting pose unique challenges and, in general, are more likely to have adverse health outcomes as a result of the ADHD (Nigg, 2013). These poor health outcomes include an association with elevated disease and death, a possible relationship to obesity, and an increased risk of accidental injury (Nigg, 2013).

Potential Impact on Communication

The National Alliance on Mental Illness (2018) notes that around two-thirds of children with ADHD also have other conditions, such as learning disabilities, emotional and behavioral disorders, anxiety, depression, obsessive-compulsive disorders, and substance abuse. These substantial comorbidities are also present in adults (Franke et al., 2018).

In a systematic meta-analytic review, Korrel and colleagues (2017) note that although the true nature of the language problems in

ADHD remains vague, some investigators support the hypothesis that children with ADHD have poorer performance on measures of overall expressive, receptive, and pragmatic language. For example, in a study by Helland, Helland, and Heimann (2014), children with ADHD performed similarly to those with specific language impairments in an overall communication measure, as well as in the pragmatic domain. According to Schreiber and colleagues, working memory is a primary impairment and these weaknesses may underlie the academic problems often seen in children with ADHD (Schreiber et al., 2014).

Several studies showed disturbances in numerous cognitive domains in adults with ADHD, including attention, executive functioning, and memory (Boonstra, Oosterlaan, Sergeant, & Buitelaar, 2005; Fuermaier et al., 2014; Fuermaier et al., 2015). Additionally, adults with ADHD obtained significantly worse results than adults with normal development on reading speed, responses to literal questions, and a cloze test (Miranda, Mercader, Fernández, & Colomer, 2017). However, adults with ADHD are reported to have good awareness of their own cognitive problems and abilities across multiple domains, despite decreased meta-cognitive abilities (Fuermaier et al., 2014). Thus, both children and adults with ADHD who are receiving services in the medical setting for a newly acquired diagnosis will require special considerations by the speech-language pathologist.

Role of the SLP

Speech-language pathologists address the language, planning and organization, attention, and social/pragmatic issues associated with the ADHD. During the evaluation of patients in the medical setting, it is important to realize that a history of premorbid ADHD may complicate the behavioral presentation of patients with a stroke, head injury, or other medical condition. It will be imperative to view the current cognitive-linguistic symptoms through the broader lens of what might be expected from someone with ADHD. Additionally, determining baseline cognitive-linguistic functioning, via self- or informant-report, will be helpful in understanding the sequelae attributed to the new medical condition.

The speech-language pathologist working in the medical setting should consult and collaborate with psychologists, psychiatrists, and others who specialize in this area for additional management. Behavioral therapy and medications can help manage and improve the symptoms of ADHD (National Alliance on Mental Illness, 2018). In a randomized control trial of cognitive behavioral therapy for ADHD in medically-treated adolescents, Sprich and colleagues demonstrated an advantage to adding cognitive behavioral therapy to medication treatment, compared to medication alone (Sprich, Safren, Finkelstein, Remmert, & Hammerness, 2016). Because of the underlying attention-deficit/hyperactivity disorder, the speech-language pathologist may need to structure the intervention differently to best support the patient. Well-established classroom strategies would likely be applicable in the medical setting as well. Paul and Norbury (2012) define categories and levels of intervention as universal, secondary (targeted), and tertiary (individualized). The universal level of intervention includes use of planners, calendars, and monitoring of organization. The secondary level of intervention includes peer-tutoring, providing choices to increase engagement, and family involvement. Tertiary level intervention includes identification of triggers, implementation of a management plan, use of a reminder systems, and encouragement of self-monitoring.

Schizophrenia and Schizoaffective Disorders

Nature of Schizophrenia and Schizoaffective Disorders

It is likely that a speech-language pathologist working in a medical setting has encountered a patient with a history of mental illness, including schizophrenia or schizoaffective disorder. Although sometimes used synonymously, they represent different disorders. According to the National Alliance on Mental Illness, schizophrenia includes delusions, hallucinations, disorganized speech, disorganized or catatonic behavior, and general apathy. Schizoaffective disorders, on the other hand, comprise all of the symptoms of schizophrenia, in addition to mood-related episodes that are either depressive in nature, manic in nature, or a combination of both.

Potential Impact on Communication/Swallowing

It is well understood that individuals with schizophrenia have impairments of language and cognition that impact their social skills and ability to participate in society. Disruption to higher-level language skills is often noted, such as difficulty with comprehension of inferred meaning, emotional prosody, discourse expression/comprehension, and pragmatic functioning (Pawelczyk, Kotlicka-Antczak, Łojek, Ruszpel, & Pawełczyk, 2018). Verbal underproductivity and disconnected speech are also common, and have been shown to negatively impact occupational and community functioning (Muralidharan, Finch, Bowie, & Harvey, 2018).

A systematic review by Joyal, Bonneau, and Fecteau (2016) noted improvements following treatment of pragmatic and discourse skills. Interestingly, the authors point out that much of the intervention with patients with schizophrenia was delivered by social workers and occupational therapists and that the expertise of the speech-language pathologist in this arena was questioned, given the psychiatric nature of the diagnosis. However, the speech-language pathologist's knowledge of language and communication makes him/her well suited for treatment in this area. Of the studies examined, the treatment approaches that yielded positive results were centered on pragmatics, social cognition, and discourse.

Although motor speech disorders are relatively uncommon in schizophrenia and schizoaffective disorders, it is likely that an affective-prosodic disturbance is present (Compton et al., 2018; Ross et al., 2001). Additionally, the neuroleptic medication used in the treatment of schizophrenia can often lead to extrapyramidal symptoms and a subsequent hypokinetic (Parkinson-like), or hyperkinetic (e.g., tardive dyskinesia) dysarthria.

Swallowing disorders are rather common. Kulkarni, Kamath, and Stewart (2017) provide an overview of swallowing problems in schizophrenia, including pathophysiology and management. They note two primary categories of swallowing problems, including those related to the illness itself that are behavioral in nature and those related to psychotropic medications. The behavioral disorders included increased rate of eating, intake of inappropriately large volumes, inadequate chewing, ingestion of nonfood items, and pocketing. Medication-related disorders included drug-induced Parkinsonism, dystonic reaction, tardive dyskinesia, xerostomia, sialorrhea, and sedation.

Role of the SLP

Schizophrenia and schizoaffective disorders often lead to communication and swallowing disorders. Working with individuals with these disorders to improve cognitive, linguistic, or swallowing skills is within the scope of practice of speech-language pathologists, as guided by the American Speech-Language-Hearing Association (ASHA, 2016). There could be a variety of reasons why a patient with this diagnosis is admitted to the medical setting, such as self-injury, abuse of alcohol or other drugs, viral hepatitis, or cardiovascular disease (Ringen, Engh, Birkenaes, Andreassen, & Andreassen, 2014; Smith, Langan, McLean, Guthrie, & Mercer, 2013). The speech-language pathologist would need to carefully parse out the deficits and determine which deficits are new for this admission or a part of the ongoing symptoms of the mental illness. For example, in an acute care setting, the speech-language pathologist might diagnosis and treat a new dysphagia, then refer back to the outpatient SLP for strategies to manage the chronic cognitive/linguistic deficits.

Given the complexity of psychiatric illnesses and medication side effects, the speech-language pathologist will need to work closely with other team members, namely the psychiatrist, psychologist, pharmacist, and the physician to best support individuals with schizophrenia (Joyal, Bonneau, & Fecteau, 2016). Improved communication, primarily via increased thought organization and enhanced pragmatic skills, would be a typical goal for the patient with schizophrenia. Clinical suggestions provided by the speech-language pathologist might include training communication partners to use simpler syntactic structure because of frequently occurring deficits in verbal working memory (Li et al., 2018). The SLP would want to ensure that the patient with schizophrenia understands the information being conveyed by medical providers. Additionally, the speech-language pathologist should also be attuned to the common, impactful side effects of neuroleptic medications, such as sedation and extrapyramidal effects (e.g., bradykinesia, dystonia, tardive dyskinesia, etc.).

Adults with mental illness showing signs of dysphagia are less likely to be referred for an instrumental swallowing assessment (Aldridge & Taylor, 2012). The role of the speech-language pathologist here may be to simply consider an instrumental swallowing assessment when dysphagia is in question for a patient with a psychiatric condition. Given the higher risk of choking in this population, a behavioral intervention approach that includes awareness training of rate and volume, verbal and written cues, diet modification, and mealtime supervision is warranted in a medical setting (Kulkarni, Kamath, & Stewart, 2017). A multidisciplinary approach to provide support to individuals with schizophrenia would be most beneficial.

Delirium

Nature of Delirium

People experiencing delirium are often present on the speech-language pathologist's caseload in a medical setting, particularly in the intensive care unit (ICU). The problems and potential complications of delirium are far-reaching. The *DSM-5* defines delirium as a disturbance of consciousness characterized by an acute onset of brain dysfunction that impacts overall cognitive functioning, attention, and thinking (American Psychiatric Association, 2013). Over 80% of patients in the ICU are reported to have delirium, yet it remains underdiagnosed (Kalbalik, Brunetti, & El-Srougy, 2014). There are many precipitating factors of delirium, as described in Table 2–2. As explained by Welch and Carson (2018), delirium may present more like a psychiatric disorder, yet is a sign of an underlying, often not yet diagnosed medical condition. Thus, the speech-language pathologist practicing in the medical setting needs to be familiar with screenings for delirium and advocate for them when appropriate. In the medical setting, it should be considered delirium until proven otherwise.

Table 2–2. Common Precipitating Factors of Delirium

Infection
Urinary tract infection
Pneumonia
Any infection, particularly with high fevers (e.g., sepsis)
Metabolic Disturbance
Hepatic failure
Chronic kidney disease
Electrolyte imbalance
Dehydration
Hypo- / hyperglycemia
Hypoxia
Vitamin Deficiency
Vitamin B12
Thiamine
Endocrine Disease
Thyroid dysfunction
Cushing's syndrome
Disorders of Excretion
Constipation (fecal impaction)
Urinary retention
Intracranial Causes
Trauma
Tumor
Abscess
Subarachnoid hemorrhage
Epilepsy
Iatrogenic Causes
Medications
Polypharmacy
Insertion of urinary catheter
Postoperative states
Substance Abuse
Alcohol intoxication or withdrawal
Barbiturate withdrawal
Pain
Any condition causing pain
Changes in Environment
For example, being admitted to hospital for an unrelated illness (especially common in patients with dementia)

Sources: Kumar et al., 2018; Raju & Coombe-Jones, 2015.

Delirium can present as three different subtypes. As described by Raju and Coombe-Jones (2015), hyperactive delirium is characterized by heightened arousal, restlessness, agitation and irritability, while hypoactive delirium is manifested as withdrawal, lethargy, and quietness. The third subtype is a mix of hyperactive and hypoactive delirium; the patient may switch back and forth between hyperactive and hypoactive states. The symptoms often fluctuate and tend to be worse at night.

The updated classification of delirium in the *DSM-5* no longer uses the term "consciousness" in its criteria, but rather focuses on cognitive functions (American Psychiatric Association, 2013). The first criterion is a disturbance in attention, which includes reduced ability to direct, focus, sustain, and shift attention, and awareness, which involves reduced orientation to the environment. The second criterion is that the disturbance develops over a short period of time and is characterized by an acute change from baseline, with fluctuations in severity over the course of a day. The third criterion includes an additional disturbance in cognitive function, such as memory, orientation, language, or perception. These disturbances cannot be better explained by a previously established or evolving neurocognitive disorder and they cannot occur in the context of a severely reduced level of arousal. The delirium must be a direct physiological consequence of another medical condition, of substance intoxication or withdrawal, of exposure to a toxin, or of multiple etiologies (European Delirium Association and American Delirium Society, 2014).

Potential Impact on Communication

Risk of long-term cognitive-communication problems is a reality with increased ICU stays, and significant efforts are being made to decrease ICU length of stay through early mobilization protocols. That is, patients are encouraged to sit at the edge of the bed, stand, get out of bed, and even ambulate. This is counter to the traditional approach of deep sedation and bed rest. Over a decade ago, it was reported by Needham (2008) that early mobilization may be the key to minimize the negative impact from bedrest. Early mobilization programs in the ICU have demonstrated feasibility, safety, and improved patient outcomes (Hashem, Nelliot, & Needham, 2016). Protocols and programs have been developed in conjunction with physical and occupational therapy. Hemodynamic stability is typically a prerequisite and, pending readiness, physical therapists and nurses would move patients from supported sitting, to sitting, to standing, to pregait activities/exercises, to ambulation (Zomorodi, Topley, & McAnaw, 2012).

The "Bringing to Light the Risk Factors and Incidences of Neuropsychological Dysfunction in ICU Survivors (BRAIN-ICU) Study," funded in part by the National Institutes of Health, concluded that a longer extent of delirium in the hospital was linked to worse global cognition and executive function scores at 3 and 12 months (Pandharipande et al., 2013). Current research appears to support the notion that patients in medical and surgical ICUs who survive critical illness are at high risk for long-term cognitive impairment (Wilcox et al., 2013).

Role of the SLP

In general, delirium is treated as a medical emergency with the focus on finding the underlying cause or causes, while ensuring the safety of the patient. The speech-language pathologist can be an integral member of the team that screens patients for delirium. During the early mobilization programs and protocols, the speech-language pathologist would often carefully coordinate their therapy schedule with physical and occupational therapy.

The prevalence of delirium in older persons in the ICU is high, particularly when they are mechanically ventilated (Kalish,

Gillham, & Unwin, 2014). The role of the speech-language pathologist in the ICU with patients with delirium can be impactful, especially for supporting communication and swallowing, and minimizing long-term cognitive impairments. Early consultation of the speech-language pathologist for weaning the patient from mechanical ventilation in order to address communication and swallowing can be critical to minimize an ICU stay and the impact of delirium. Johnson et al. (2018) recently published the validation of a postextubation dysphagia screening tool for particular use with patients after prolonged endotracheal intubation in the ICU. Additionally, they note the importance of speech-language pathologists and nurses working collaboratively in an effort to minimize delays or referrals. Furthermore, use of a speaking valve might be indicated for some patients, and would warrant an evaluation for readiness by the speech-language pathologist under close monitoring.

Speech-language pathologists also have a role in the education of the family, including how to gently redirect and provide orientation information to the patient. Orientation may be enhanced by sufficient lighting and clear signage. The speech-language pathologist should also explain their role in the patient's health care to help keep the patient oriented. They can advocate for reduced noise/distractions in the patient's room, and should make sure the patient stays hydrated. The needs of patients with delirium are considerable and speech-language pathologists are continuing to develop more of a presence in their care.

CARDIAC AND RESPIRATORY DISORDERS

Doreen Kelly Izaguirre

Cardiac, cardiovascular, and respiratory disorders comprise a substantial portion of the caseload for many speech-language pathologists in a medical setting. A solid understanding of the systems, conditions, and treatments related to cardiovascular and respiratory disease, as well as a familiarity with medical terminology for this population, will be critical. In the medical setting, speech-language pathologists will frequently receive consults to evaluate and treat patients with chronic obstructive pulmonary disease, acute respiratory failure, and heart failure, including those with ventricular assistive devices, to list a few.

Chronic Obstructive Pulmonary Disease (COPD)

Nature of COPD

Chronic obstructive pulmonary disease is a term that refers to a group of lung diseases, including chronic bronchitis, emphysema, and asthma. Chronic bronchitis is an inflammation of the bronchial airways in the lungs. This inflammation and irritation limits airflow and makes breathing difficult. In emphysema, the small and delicate alveoli are damaged, making it hard to get oxygen in and carbon dioxide out. Asthma is a type of bronchial airway obstruction characterized by airway tightening and swelling.

The ICD-9 uses COPD as the umbrella term to capture this group of frequently overlapping chronic lung diseases. However, in the ICD-10, these diseases are now referred to as chronic lower respiratory disease or CLRD (World Health Organization, 2014). Generally speaking, both COPD and CLRD are characterized by shortness of breath secondary to some form of airway obstruction (World Health Organization, 2014). CLRDs affect approximately 1 in 12 people worldwide, and are a major cause of morbidity and mortality (Oelsner et al., 2016). In 2017, the Centers for Disease Control (CDC) listed CLRD as

the fourth leading cause of death behind diseases of the heart, malignant neoplasms, and unintentional injuries.

Potential Impact on Communication/Swallowing

As noted by Cvejic and Bardin (2018), problems with swallowing, including aspiration, have long been recognized in COPD, yet remain poorly understood. Impaired coordination of breathing and swallowing, in particular, often leads to dysphagia in individuals with COPD (Steidl et al., 2015). Given the complex relationship of breathing and swallowing, objective instrumentation is recommended to understand breathing and swallowing coordination, as well as the pharyngeal phase physiology, airway closure and timing, and presence of residue. Instrumental assessment for swallowing often includes videofluoroscopic swallow study (VFSS) and fiberoptic endoscopic evaluation of swallowing (FEES).

COPD causes symptoms of breathlessness and breathing discomfort (dyspnea), which limits daily activities and reduces quality of life (Xu, He, Han, Pan, & Cao, 2017). Speech can be particularly affected during conversation, speaking loudly, speaking on the telephone, talking in a noisy place, and singing (Binazzi et al., 2011), particularly in the later stages of COPD/CLRD. Intervention will be required to assure the patient has the ability to communicate wants, needs, and ideas in a variety of settings to maximize quality of life. Considerations may also be needed for a functional communication system after discharge from the medical setting if safety is a concern.

Role of the SLP

The role of the speech-language pathologist is often twofold with individuals with CLRD.

Because breathing and swallowing overlap physically and functionally, an understanding of the coordination of both systems is vital to being an effective clinician with this population. Dysphagia-oriented treatment consists mostly of behavioral strategies during meal times, such as small bites and sips, double swallow, and rest breaks throughout the meal, to list a few. Working closely with the multidisciplinary team, including the physician, pulmonologist, occupational therapist, and dietitian is important. Patients with breathing difficulty that may include increased respiratory rate and shortness of breath, may benefit from having smaller meals throughout the day to safely meet their nutrition and hydration needs.

The speech-language pathologist can also support speech production by training proper phrase length and perhaps recommending amplification for those with decreased volume. Some patients with more advanced COPD/CLRD are at high risk for major complications and may require more aggressive management for pulmonary hygiene and gas exchange. These include tracheostomy tubes, mechanical ventilation, and noninvasive ventilation. These approaches are further discussed in another section of this chapter.

Acute Respiratory Failure (ARF)

Nature of Acute Respiratory Failure (ARF)

Acute respiratory failure is a sudden, life threatening condition characterized by trouble breathing, markedly low levels of oxygen, and extremely high levels of carbon dioxide in the blood (Golper, Klaben, & Miller, 2019). Speech-language pathologists in the medical setting often work with patients in acute respiratory failure, typically through clinical and instrumental swallowing evaluations. Because of the significant breathing problems

of patients with ARF, the speech-language pathologist will need to have extensive knowledge of tracheostomy tubes, mechanical ventilation, and non-invasive ventilation to competently evaluate and develop an intervention plan for the patient.

Potential Impact on Communication/Swallowing

The swallowing and speech functioning of the patient in acute respiratory failure is highly dependent upon the patient presentation and overall severity level. Pulmonary/respiratory stability will take precedent over speech and swallowing functioning. The speech-language pathologist would receive a consult to evaluate dysphagia when the patient is considered stable; Figure 2–1 provides a standard consultation protocol. Dysphagia is reported to occur in 20% (Macht, White, & Moss, 2014) to 60% (Lynch et al., 2017) of ARF survivors. Unfortunately, many patients who survive ARF must also cope with debilitating consequences of their critical illness, including neuromuscular weakness, cognitive dysfunction, and symptoms of depression and anxiety (Herridge et al., 2011).

Role of the SLP

In the intensive care setting, acute changes in a patient's status may take place minute-by-minute, or hour-by-hour. In the general medical and rehabilitation settings, the patient is more stable and these acute changes happen less frequently. A multidisciplinary approach to the management of patients with ARF is recommended. Following a five-year investigation, Prohaska et al. (2017) revealed patterns of underutilization of physical therapy, occupational therapy, and speech-language pathology services, especially in the critically ill population with ARF receiving mechanical ventilation. The speech-language pathologist

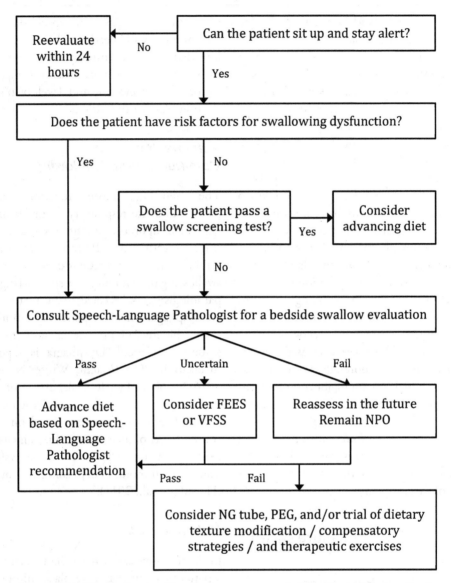

Figure 2–1. Diagnostic algorithm for the assessment of swallowing dysfunction in patients recovering from critical illness. *Note.* FEES = fiberoptic endoscopic evaluation of swallowing; NG = nasogastric; NPO = translates to "nothing by mouth"; PEG = percutaneous endoscopic gastrostomy; VFSS = videoflouroscopic swallow study. *Source:* Reprinted from M. Macht, D. White, and M. Moss, (2014). Swallowing Dysfunction After Critical Illness. *Chest, 146*(6), 1681–1689, with permission from Elsevier.

should establish a strong working relationship with the respiratory care providers to determine readiness and timing of interventions to increase communication and initiate swallowing, under the direction of the physician. The role of the speech-language pathologist may also include patient advocacy (timing of speaking valve readiness; alternative-augmentative communication) or advocacy for their value-added service in the ICU.

Heart Failure and Ventricular Assistive Devices (VAD)

Nature of Heart Failure and Ventricular Assistive Devices (VAD)

Heart failure is a major health problem associated with disease and death (Giamouzis et al., 2011). There are several heart failure stages, as described by the American Heart Association (2018):

- **Stage A:** Presence of heart failure risk factors but no heart disease and no symptoms.
- **Stage B:** Heart disease is present (structural changes in heart), but there are no symptoms.
- **Stage C:** Structural heart disease is present and symptoms have occurred.
- **Stage D:** Presence of advanced heart disease with continued heart failure symptoms requiring aggressive medical therapy.

Heart failure occurs when the cardiac muscle becomes too weak or too stiff and fails to pump the blood throughout the body as it should. This condition results from a variety of diseases and conditions, such as coronary artery disease and high blood pressure. Heart failure can be acute, or present as a chronic illness that will get worse over time without management. According to the National Heart, Lung, and Blood Institute (2018), the goal of heart failure management is often to slow down or stop the progression into the later stages of heart failure. The options progress from lifestyle and medication management, to surgery, to assistive devices, and/or ultimately transplant.

When stopping the progression of heart failure is not possible and management via medications or lifestyle changes has been unsuccessful, other options are explored. Technology is one consideration, such as ventricular assistive devices (VAD), with left ventricular assistive devices (LVAD) being most common. Ventricular assistive devices (VAD) are transplantable devices that help to support the function of the left, right, or both ventricles, or lower chambers, in the heart. They pump blood from one main chamber to the body or the other side of the heart. These devices provide short-term support for patients who are awaiting cardiac transplantation, or long-term support for patients who may not be candidates for a transplant. They are an option for patients in late stage heart failure, including congestive heart failure, and are often used in patients with high CHADS risk scores (a system for stratifying risk of stroke; Gage et al., 2001) from congestive heart failure, hypertension, age ≥75, diabetes mellitus, and prior stroke. Use of VADs typically occurs in the latest stage of heart failure, or Stage D.

Potential Impact on Commuincation/Swallowing

Some of the signs and symptoms of heart failure will impact swallowing and interfere with cognitive-communication skills. These include fatigue, shortness of breath, difficulty sleeping, pulmonary edema (excess fluid in the lungs), pleural effusion (excess fluid around the lungs), abdominal swelling, and fluid overload (National Heart, Lung, and Blood Institute, 2018; Theander et al., 2014). Cognitive impairment is frequent in patients with heart failure. Bhat, Yost, and Mahoney (2015) note the prevalence of cognitive impairment ranges from 25% to 75%, citing poor cerebral perfusion as a primary possible reason. Two large multicenter studies have also indicated that cognitive impairment in patients with heart failure is associated with a sixfold increase in functional disability (Bhat, Yost, & Mahoney, 2015; Zuccalà et al., 2001; Zuccalà et al., 2003). The cognitive impairments often seen in patients in heart failure involve learning, delayed recall, attention, executive function, psychomotor speed, and working memory, with less of an impact on language and visuospatial skills (Leto & Feloa, 2014).

Role of the SLP

The speech-language pathologist working with cardiac patients will need to understand cardiac parameters and associated problems that may impact assessment and intervention. One parameter, expressed as a percentage, is ejection fraction (EF). Ejection fraction refers to how well the left or right ventricle drives blood with each contraction. The main chamber of the heart is the left ventricle, so typically the percentage is referencing the amount of blood that is being pumped out of the left ventricle (Cleveland Clinic, 2018). Guidelines for heart function provided by the Cleveland Clinic include normal pumping ability at 55% to 70%, slightly below normal at 40% to 54%, moderately below normal at 35% to 39%, and severely below normal at less than 35%.

The speech-language pathologist will also often conduct evaluation and treatment of cognitive-communication deficits, including how these deficits impact patient safety and independence. For those patients who are candidates for VAD placement, early assessment, even pretransplantation when available, as well as cognitive-communication intervention posttransplantation, can be effective (Bhat, Yost, & Mahoney, 2015).

Improved cardiac output, especially in the early stages of heart failure, can have a positive impact on a patient's cognitive status (Leto & Feola, 2014). There is preliminary evidence to suggest that the placement of a ventricular assistive device can result in improved cognitive skills as well as reduced depression in patients in heart failure (Bhat,

Yost, & Mahoney, 2015). In those patients with VAD transplants, there is a substantial amount of new learning that is required posttransplantation. The speech-language pathologist can implement a functional approach to rehabilitation that includes memory strategy training and extensive family/caregiver training.

HEAD AND NECK SURGERY

Matina Balou

The head and neck region involves a number of complex neurovascular structures responsible for respiration, phonation, articulation, resonance, and swallowing. When treating head and neck tumors, the goal is to preserve the functionality of those structures surrounding the tumor. However, treatment modalities for head and neck cancer, which include surgery, radiation, and concurrent chemotherapy and radiation, can impact both the anatomy as well as the physiology of the muscles involved in speech and swallowing (Arrese & Hutcheson, 2018).

Dysphagia is sometimes present pretreatment, and the severity of the dysphagia has been shown to correlate with disease stage (Pauloski et al., 2000; Starmer, Gourin, Lua, & Burkhead, 2011; van der Molen et al., 2009). It has been estimated that 38% of patients with head and neck cancer initially present with swallowing impairment (Salama et al., 2008). Interference of the normal physiology of swallowing may be due to tumor invasion of surrounding structures or the tumor itself.

The management of speech and swallowing disorders is crucial to optimize the quality of life before and after treatment of individuals with head and neck cancer. Speech-language pathologists play a vital role in both inpatient and outpatient settings to optimize communication and to ensure safe swallowing (Hansen,

Chenoweith, Thompson, & Strouss, 2018). Early involvement by the SLP facilitates patient compliance and ultimately improves short- and long-term outcomes for the patient (Lewin, Teng, & Kotz, 2016). Speech and swallow exercises are often started immediately, even before the cancer treatment. During these pretreatment sessions, the plan for speech, voice, and swallow rehabilitation posttreatment is reviewed, along with the importance of the patient's active participation in the treatment planning and program (Kotz et al., 2012).

The severity of posttreatment dysphagia and speech difficulty is directly related to the site of lesion and the cancer treatment modality (Pauloski et al., 2000). Multimodality therapies are common practice for treatment of head and neck cancer for approximately 80% of all patients. Surgery is usually considered in order to excise the tumor, and typically results in abnormal deglutition and disrupted speech due to loss of tissue. Radiation and chemotherapy can also have detrimental effects on swallowing (Granell et al., 2012) and speech (Jacobi, van der Molen, Huiskens, van Rossum, & Hilgers, 2010).

Lip Surgery

Cancer of the lip is the most common malignant tumor affecting the head and neck region (Zerninsky, Zini, & Sgan-Cohen, 2010). In some ways, its clinical behavior is similar to that of skin cancer in terms of treatment options. The lips are an often overlooked site for nonmelanoma skin cancers, including the two most common skin cancers, basal and squamous cell. Incidence rates are around 12.7 per 100,000 in North America, 12 per 100,000 in Europe, and 13.5 per 100,000 in Oceania (Zerninsky, Zini, & Sgan-Cohen, 2010).

Early stage lip cancer can be treated equally well by surgery or radiation therapy,

and neck dissection is generally not performed unless there is suspicion of the presence of cancer in cervical lymph nodes. Small lesions are managed by simple surgical excision and primary closure, whereas larger lesions of the lip require more consideration with regard to reconstruction techniques (Kerawala, Roques, Jeannon, & Bisase, 2016). The functional outcome of the repair with regard to lip sensitivity and muscle function also needs to be taken into consideration. The primary aim of surgery in any oral cavity cancer is tumor resection with cancer-free margins of 1 cm (Gerber, Gengler, Gratz, & Kruse, 2011). A histopathological margin of less than 5 mm leads to further surgery or adjuvant radiotherapy. "Close margin" is a term used by pathologists that implies that tumor cells are lying in the vicinity of excised margin (varies anywhere between 1 mm and 5 mm) (Paxton, 2013). The assessment and treatment of the tumor is largely based upon clinical and radiological findings (for example, patient symptoms, tumor invasion to nearby tissues seen radiographically; Brown et al., 2005). Following surgery, the medical team would address any remaining cancer cells with chemotherapy and/or radiotherapy (Paxton, 2013).

The subsequent loss of the upper or lower lip due to surgery may lead to loss of oral competence, oral bolus control, reduced oral bolus preparation, and anterior loss of bolus. Microstomia, which is a reduction in the size of the oral cavity as a result of the labial reconstruction, may also affect bolus introduction to the mouth (Leonard & Kendall, 2014).

Tongue Surgery

In patients with intraoral cancers, dysphagia is caused by loss or dysfunction of swallowing-related structures, limited or inadequate movement of the remaining structures, and/or sensory damage to the tongue, oral mucosa, and pharynx. The degree of dysphagia depends mostly on the location and the extent of the tongue resection (McConnel et al., 1994). Namaki and colleagues (2011) reported that patients experienced dysphagia when they had a glossectomy involving more than 50% of their tongue.

The extent of the dysphagia may not be ascertained immediately postoperation. Patient-reported swallowing outcomes revealed more difficulties with swallowing at 1 month postoperation compared with baseline (Dzioba et al., 2017). However, by 6 months postoperation, the swallowing difficulties can dissipate.

Patients treated for oral tongue cancer may also experience long-term speech problems (Dwivedi et al., 2012; Rinkel, Verdonck-de Leeuw, van Reij, Aaronson, & Leemans, 2008; Rinkel, Verdonck-de Leeuw, de Bree, Aaronson, & Leemans, 2015). Postoperative defects in tongue size and form as a result of glossectomy can cause sound distortions and have a detrimental impact on speech intelligibility. Loss of intelligibility reduces the effectiveness of communication and can result in reticence or avoidance regarding social situations, thus impacting the patient's quality of life (Constantinescu, Rieger, Winget, Paulsen, & Seikaly, 2017; Stone, Langguth, Woo, Chen, & Prince, 2014). Dwivedi and colleagues (2012), in a cross-sectional study of patients with head and neck cancer (average of 78 months postsurgery), concluded that speech impairment may be present many years following surgical intervention.

Surgery of the Oropharynx

The oropharynx consists of the tongue base, the faucial arches, tonsils and the tonsillar fosa, the retromolar trigone, soft palate, and the pharyngeal walls of the superior and lateral pharynx (Groher & Crary, 2010). The swallowing impairments that can emerge following oropharyngeal surgery include decreased pharyngeal stripping wave (pressure generated by the constrictor muscles), aspiration, nasal regurgitation, and reduced upper esophageal sphincter opening. Extensive surgery to excise the cancer may subsequently require reconstruction surgery as well. Khariwala and colleagues (2007) reported that the most difficult subsites to reconstruct were tongue defects, which were strongly correlated with poor swallowing outcomes. Flaps used for tissue reconstruction may also contribute to poor movement of oropharyngeal muscles.

On the other hand, the use of radiation and chemotherapy as a primary treatment for oropharyngeal cancer has been beneficial in sparing the side effects of surgery and removal of tissues and musculature involved in swallowing. However, organ preservation does not necessarily mean preservation of function. A substantial body of evidence suggests that patients receiving nonsurgical treatment for oropharyngeal cancer are experiencing acute toxicities and long-term alteration of swallow function (Starmer et al., 2014).

Speech can also be detrimentally affected by oropharygeal cancer, as the range of movement, strength, and accuracy of the articulators can be altered by the cancer or its treatment (Saravanan, Ranganathan, Gandhi, & Jaya, 2016). Persistent, severe speech problems have been associated with radiation therapy, late stage tumors (stage III–IV), and tumors located on the floor of the mouth (Suarez-Cunqueiro et al., 2008).

Surgery of the Hypopharynx and Larynx

The hypopharynx is a tube-like structure that includes the pyriform sinuses, pharyngeal walls, and postcricoid area. Early hypopharyngeal cancer can be removed with less invasive surgical procedures. For example, in endoscopic transoral resection, a surgeon removes cancerous tissue with an endoscope while viewing the anatomy of the area through a microscope. Surgeons may also perform robotic-assisted surgery to remove hypopharyngeal tumors. Usually, hypopharyngeal tumors are advanced at the time of diagnosis because there are no significant overt symptoms and, therefore, they may require extensive surgery (Groher & Crary, 2010). If cancer has spread to other parts of the pharynx, surgeons may remove all or part of the pharynx with a procedure called pharyngectomy. If the larynx is affected, surgeons may perform a laryngectomy. Surgery also involves reconstruction to restore functional continuity of the aerodigestive tract (Logemann, Paoloski, Rademaker, & Colangelo, 1997; Patel et al., 2010).

The importance of speech and swallow function with respect to quality of life is well known (Logemann et al., 1997). These functions can be drastically affected due to the anatomical changes to the pharynx and larynx following surgical resection. Laryngectomy directly impacts the ability to communicate due to the altered airway and removal of the larynx, leaving the patient with the inability to produce voice. Patients must learn to communicate in new ways; a range of speech rehabilitation techniques are available to patients following total laryngectomy. As the larynx is completely removed, the communication options are limited to: (a) nonvocal communication; (b) esophageal speech; (c) use of an artificial larynx; or (d) tracheoesophageal speech (Sharpe et al., 2018). Most patients undergo placement of a trachea-esophageal puncture with insertion of a tracheoesophageal prosthesis. Surgically, a small opening is created between the trachea and esophagus, and a voice prosthesis valve is placed in the opening. When the stoma is blocked, air is directed through the prosthesis, which then vibrates the pharyngoesophageal segment in

the throat. The one-way nature of the voice prosthesis prevents food and drink from passing to the airway. To achieve voice, patients can occlude the stoma with their thumb or use a hands-free device to direct air through the prosthesis for speech (Sharpe et al., 2018).

Base of the Skull Surgery

Due to the complexity of skull base anatomy, lesions involving the skull base can result in a number of motor and sensory impairments. Understanding the lower cranial nerves assists with identifying the potential deficits that can result from the tumor itself and subsequent treatment (Peterson & Fenn, 2005). For instance, the glossopharyngeal nerve is a mixed sensory and motor nerve. The pharyngeal branches of this nerve innervate the stylopharyngeus muscle (elevates the pharynx during swallowing and speech), and receives sensory information from several structures, including the tonsils, anterior/posterior tonsillar pillars, and posterior one-third of the tongue. Because it provides taste and sensation for the posterior tongue, glossopharyngeal nerve deficits may impact swallowing sensation (Peterson & Fenn, 2005). The impact to speech is less well understood because it becomes intertwined with the more substantial vagus nerve.

The vagus nerve is the longest and most complex of the cranial nerves. Vagus nerve deficits often result in dysphagia and dysarthria. It has three primary branches related to speech and swallowing, which influence the function of the larynx (recurrent laryngeal nerve, superior laryngeal nerve) and soft palate (pharyngeal nerve). Unilateral disruption to the recurrent laryngeal nerve results in a weak, breathy voice, and problems swallowing with risk of aspiration. Because of the difficulty in adjusting laryngeal resistance with incomplete glottic closure, patients often feel short of breath (Woodson, 1993). Bilateral lesions of the recurrent laryngeal nerve will lead to similar, but exacerbated, speech and swallowing impairments. High vagal lesions typically result in failure of coordination of the oral and oropharyngeal phases of swallowing, with reduced opening and relaxation of the upper esophageal sphincter, and with hypopharyngeal residue in the pyriform sinuses and overflow into the larynx (Jennings, Siroky, & Jackson, 1992). Disruption to the pharyngeal branch can lead to hypernasality and nasal emission.

The hypoglossal nerve innervates almost all of the muscles of the tongue. Thus, hypoglossal nerve involvement by a skull base lesion results in dysarthric speech and oral-phase dysphagia. If the lesion is isolated to the hypoglossal nerve, the deficits may be compensated with swallowing and articulatory therapy (Peterson & Fenn, 2005).

Anterior Cervical Discectomy and Fusion (ACDF)

Anterior Cervical Discectomy and Fusion (ACDF) is a surgical procedure to correct pain, weakness, or numbness associated with herniated discs and/or degenerative disc disease. Unfortunately, a significant proportion (6.5% to 71%) (Bazaz, Lee, & Yoo, 2002; Frempong-Boadu et al., 2002; Martin, Neary, & Diamant, 1997; Rihn, Kane, Albert, Vaccaro, & Hilibrand, 2011; Smith-Hammond et al., 2004) of individuals experience swallowing impairment post-ACDF. Dysphagia can cause reductions in quality-of-life but also can have more dire consequences, such as malnutrition, dehydration, and aspiration pneumonia. For patients undergoing ACDF surgery, the incidence of postoperative radiographic swallowing abnormalities, for those who did not have dysphagia pre-operatively, is reported to be 67% (Frempong-Boadu et al., 2002).

Female gender and surgery on multiple cervical vertebrae have been defined as important risk factors in the development of postoperative dysphagia (Lee, Bazaz, Furey, & Yoo, 2007; Sagi, Beutler, Carroll, & Connolly, 2002).

Questions still exist about the relationship between prevertebral soft tissue swelling and dysphagia. Kepler and colleagues (2012) performed a radiographic analysis of patients who underwent anterior ACDF surgery to investigate this relationship. The study found no correlation between soft-tissue swelling, measured by the anterior cervical soft-tissue shadow width on lateral cervical radiographs, and the extent of dysphagia, measured by results of a dysphagia questionnaire. However, a limitation of this study was that it did not include diagnostic testing to measure the severity of dysphagia, where aspiration is often silent or undetected.

The majority of studies utilize patient report through nonvalidated questionnaires, whereas only a limited number use gold-standard videofluoroscopic imaging. Further, variation in the literature stems from differences with respect to the timing of assessing swallowing impairment postsurgery. There are likely at least two independent contributing factors to developing dysphagia following ACDF surgery. First, many patients will experience significant postsurgical edema that is thought to contribute to acute disruption of swallowing function. This edema appears to reduce pharyngeal stripping and epiglottic inversion. which manifests in postswallow residue (Leonard & Belafsky, 2011). Second, injury to specific cranial and spinal nerves during ACDF surgery has the potential to impact swallowing function (Haller, Iwanik, & Shen, 2011). According to Lee and colleagues, structures known to be at risk are the glossopharyngeal and hypoglossal nerves, the superior laryngeal nerve, the recurrent laryngeal nerve and vagus trunk at lower cervical areas, and the cricopharyngeus. Although neurologic injury is certainly not expected in all cases of ACDF surgery, some amount of postsurgical edema is to be expected in the vast majority of cases. A particular challenge to understanding the pathophysiology of dysphagia post-ACDF is differentiating disruption to swallowing function as the result of edema from injury to the cranial nerves that are at risk during the ACDF procedure.

ESOPHAGEAL DISORDERS

Matina Balou

In esophageal dysphagia, patients often complain of difficulty swallowing and of food "sticking" in the throat or upper chest several seconds after swallowing. This contrasts with patients with oropharyngeal dysphagia, who present with symptoms such as coughing, choking, nasal regurgitation, and tracheobronchial aspiration (Hirano & Kahrilas, 2012). There are numerous causes of esophageal dysphagia; differential diagnosis will involve a multidisciplinary team effort, careful patient history, review of symptoms and medications, a physical examination, as well as an instrumental examination. Esophageal dysphagia can be caused by structural/mechanical issues that create pressure or narrowing from inside the esophagus (e.g., a mucosal ring or a tumor), or from outside the esophagus (e.g., lung cancer). It can also be caused by motor issues such as achalasia, an esophageal motility disorder, or gastroesophageal reflux disease. With the aging population in the United States, along with the increased prevalence of obesity and gastroesophageal reflux disease, health care providers will increasingly encounter older patients with esophageal disease and complaints of dysphagia (Aslam & Vaezi, 2013).

Gastroesophageal Reflux Disease (GERD)

Gastroesophageal reflux (GER) is defined as the retrograde flow of acid, pepsin, and bile from the stomach to the esophagus through the lower esophageal sphincter (LES). The physiologic reflux is usually brief and is not accompanied by symptoms, and therefore, is not always pathologic. However, when the LES relaxations are prolonged and frequent, and the gastric contents escape the LES, typical symptoms such as heartburn, regurgitation and esophageal dysphagia may occur. When symptomatic signs of tissue injury are manifest, it is referred to as gastroesophageal reflux disease (GERD). In the United States, up to 25% of adults experience heartburn at least once per month and 4% to 7% report daily heartburn (Vaezi, Hicks, Abelson, & Richter, 2003). GERD has been estimated to affect more than 59 million Americans and up to 50% of the patients with GERD suffer from dysphagia (Belafsky & Rees Lintzenich, 2014).

Individuals may also experience laryngopharyngeal reflux (LPR), which occurs when gastric contents escape through the upper esophageal sphincter and reach the laryngeal level, resulting in frequent throat clearing/coughing, hoarseness, and globus sensation (Koufman, Aviv, Casiano, & Shaw, 2002). Globus pharyngeus, or globus sensation, is one of the most common symptoms leading to a referral for a swallow evaluation to rule out oropharyngeal dysphagia. It is a high recurrence symptom with poor cure rate and relief (Koufman et al., 2002). Pharyngeal dryness, tightness, burning, itchiness, dysphagia, obstruction, and foreign body sensation are some of the most common complaints related to LPR (Ding et al., 2017). Patients with LPR usually deny events of coughing and choking during meals and have more complaints about solids but not liquids.

Presence of LPR has been associated with the development of chronic laryngitis and dysphonia as it is a chronic, local irritant (Tasli, Eser, Basik, & Birkent, 2018). Tissue changes and alterations of both Reinke's space, as well as lubrication of the free edge of the vocal folds, are some of the mechanisms explaining the voice quality changes (Naunheim & Carroll, 2017). Benign lesions of the vocal folds, including nodules, polyps, contact laryngeal ulcers, granulomas, or pseudosulcus, are some of the etiologies for patients' dysphonia (Naunheim & Carroll, 2017). Although LPR is common, its diagnosis is not easy because its symptoms are indistinct and the laryngeal findings are not always correlated with symptom severity. According to American Academy of Otolaryngology, Head & Neck Surgery (2013), some patients with LPR may or may not experience classic symptoms of heartburn. Some usual symptoms related to either GERD or LPR are:

- Heartburn
- Belching
- Regurgitation
- Frequent throat clearing or coughing
- Excess mucus
- A bitter taste
- A sensation of burning or throat soreness
- Something "stuck" or a "lump" in the back of the throat
- Hoarseness or change in voice
- Difficulty swallowing
- Drainage down the back of the nose (postnasal drip)
- Choking episodes (can sometimes awaken from sleep)

Antireflux therapy with proton pump inhibitors (PPI) is the most common treatment. After 4 weeks of PPI, dysphagia is usually resolved. Changing lifestyle and dietary modification to reduce reflux may minimize reflux in some cases. Patients may need to visit an otolaryngologist and/or a gastroenterologist, depending on the symptoms.

Esophageal Motility Disorders

Esophageal-based dysphagia may affect the oral and pharyngeal stages of swallowing, and therefore, it is important to be aware of the characteristics and symptoms. Frequently, patients experience symptoms of chest pain, dysphagia, and regurgitation. Dysphagia symptoms usually appear after the swallow or after the meal. The dysphagia is thought to be caused by intrinsic structural pathology or disruption in normal motility (Johnston, 2017). The major motility disorders are summarized in Table 2–3, and could also include ineffective esophageal motility, or disorders of peristalsis (Boo, Chik, Ngiu, Lim, & Jarmin, 2018).

A clinical history and physical exam of the patient is the best first step to determine presence of oropharyngeal versus esophageal dysphagia, asking questions regarding timing of the symptom in regards to drinking/eating, swallow initiation, regurgitation, throat clearing or coughing, and presence of repetitive swallowing (Cook, 2008).

Esophageal manometry has historically been used to diagnose motility disorders of the esophagus and, specifically, intraluminal pressures and coordination of muscular contractions within the esophagus. Recent technological advances with this procedure have made it possible to obtain accurate manometric profiles of the esophageal pressures and durations of events associated with the pharynx and UES, as well as the esophagus (Hatlebakk et al., 1998; Hila, Castell, & Castell, 2001). Nowadays, pressure sensors in high-resolution

Table 2–3. Major Types of Motility Disorders

Disorder	Cause
Achalasia	Disruption of the lower esophageal sphincter (LES) in the context of absent peristalsis
Spastic esophageal motility disorder	Diffuse esophageal spasm (DES), nutcracker esophagus, and hypertensive LES
Nonspecific esophageal motility disorder	Inefficient esophageal motility
Secondary esophageal motility disorders	Scleroderma, diabetes mellitus, alcohol consumption, psychiatric disorders, presbyesophagus

esophageal manometry (HREM) are located 1 cm apart, compared to 4 to 5 cm in conventional manometry, allowing HREM to become the most sensitive test to diagnose esophageal motility disorders (Bredenoord et al., 2012).

Multichannel intraluminal electrical impedance (MII) measurement has provided a way of defining bolus movement and esophageal clearance in conjunction with HREM. Because HREM can provide information regarding bolus flow in the esophagus, MII can differentiate the intraluminal air (which exhibits high impedance), from liquid (which exhibits low impedance). Validation studies have verified that MII measurement has high sensitivity and accuracy for detecting intra-esophageal bolus movement and monitoring reflux (Gyawali et al., 2013). A small pH catheter is passed through one side of patient's nose and is advanced into the esophagus. The catheter remains in place for 24 hours and is attached to a small recording device that is secured around the waist of the patient.

Upper Esophageal Sphincter (UES) Dysfunction

Cricopharyngeus muscle dysfunction is a common cause of dysphagia. It is an essential component of the pharyngoesophageal segment (PES) and is responsible for preventing the ingestion of air during respiration and post-swallow regurgitation of esophageal contents into the pharynx. The PES is a manometric, high-pressure zone extending 3 to 5 cm from the hypopharynx to the cervical esophagus. Dysphagia is a result of obstruction, reduced relaxation and opening, decreased hyolaryngeal elevation, or ineffective pharyngeal propulsive forces (Kuhn & Belafsky, 2013).

To swallow safely and efficiently, muscles of the tongue and pharynx must create sufficient pressures to propel the bolus through the pharynx while maintaining opening of the UES, allowing the bolus to move into the esophagus (Castell & Castell, 1997). Impairment in the timing of oropharyngeal events, the magnitude of pharyngeal propulsive force, or the extent of UES relaxation and opening can lead to varying amounts of pharyngeal residue and possible airway invasion.

Pharyngeal constriction against an obstructed pharyngoesophageal segment can lead to the development of a dilated, weak pharynx and Zenker's diverticulum (Allen, White, Leonard, & Belafsky, 2010; Belafsky, Rees, Allen, & Leonard, 2010). Zenker's diverticulum is an outpouching of mucosa and submucosa through Killian triangle, defined by the inferior constrictor muscle and the cricopharyngeal muscle (Jones et al., 2016). Some available surgical and nonsurgical treatment options to improve PES function include diet modification, swallowing exercises, botulinum toxin injection, dilation and endoscopic/open myotomy, (a laparoscopic surgical procedure) (Kuhn & Belafsky, 2013).

Videofluoroscopy is the gold standard diagnostic modality that enables visualization of the biomechanics of the oropharyngeal swallow in relation to bolus flow. Measures of structural movements and the timing and duration of those movements can be obtained, as well as the effects of those movements on food and liquid being swallowed. What cannot be assessed from videofluoroscopy are measures of pharyngeal swallowing pressures and relaxation of pressure within the upper esophageal sphincter (UES). Such pressure changes are critical to proper and safe swallowing. However, technology has enabled clinicians to use manometry and videofluoroscopic swallow study (VFSS) simultaneously (i.e., videomanometry) to obtain information about pressures in the pharynx and UES while the biomechanics of swallowing function are observed (Bülow, Olsson & Ekberg, 1999; Olsson, Castell, Johnston, Ekberg, & Castell, 1997; Olsson, Nilsson, & Ekberg, 1994; Pauloski et al., 2008). For this purpose, "videomanometry" offers a combined qualitative assessment of bolus transport achieved by VFSS with the quantitative mapping of pharyngeal and UES pressures, durations, and coordination timings obtained by the pharyngeal and esophageal manometry.

Olsson and colleagues (1994) investigated the usefulness of videomanometry in the routine radiologic evaluation of dysphagia. First, the patients underwent VFSS alone to determine swallowing function. Then, simultaneous VFSS and solid-state intraluminal manometry was performed in 30 individuals with a mean age of 55 years. The authors reported sixteen patients had a normal VFSS, but five of these patients had pathologic findings with videomanometry. High contraction amplitudes and increased resting pressures in the UES were present in those patients. Thus, the authors concluded that videomanometry can add information regarding swallowing function that is not obtainable by either of the two methods alone. Similar findings were reported by Olsson and Ekberg (2005) who found that a combined approach was best for patients with a posterior cricopharyngeal (CP) bar (poor relaxation of the sphincter and muscle hypertrophy). That is, patients with a CP bar exhibited normal UES relaxation and resting pressures but abnormally wide superior and inferior segments of UES activity providing low contraction pressures during videomanometry.

The presence and cause of pharyngeal residue in the valleculae and/or in the pyriform sinuses is also important to note. Residue increases risk of aspiration after the swallow (Groher & Crary, 2010; Ekberg & Wahlgren, 1985). Neither VFSS nor manometry alone can effectively determine the complex causes of residue in the pharynx. VFSS provides visualization of the residue, as well as movements of the epiglottis and hyolaryngeal mechanism that can facilitate or impede bolus flow. Manometry provides information regarding any decrease in pharyngeal pressure or delays in UES relaxation that could result in residue. Simultaneous VFSS and solid-state intraluminal manometry have been utilized to verify the association between defective elevation of the larynx and pharyngeal residue, as well as decreased UES opening and pharyngeal residue (Olsson et al., 1997). Therefore, even if the role of the speech-language pathologist is not to treat esophageal dysphagia, it is important to know how esophageal disorders may affect pharyngeal and oropharyngeal stages of swallowing and to be able to refer the patient to the appropriate health care provider.

CASE STUDIES

Case 1

ZJ is a 17-year-old male who was hit by a drunk driver while he was driving home after a party. Glasgow Coma Scale on scene was 5 (Eye opening: 2; Verbal response: 1; Motor response: 2). He was intubated on scene and remained in a coma for 7 days post injury. MRI revealed bifrontal and occipital cerebral contusions along with diffuse axonal injury. Significant swelling of the brain was noted and neurosurgery completed a decompressive craniectomy to relieve the pressure and prevent herniation. After ZJ emerged from coma, seizure activity was noted for which antiseizure medication was initiated. He also required a tracheostomy after failed attempts at extubation. Over the course of several sessions, the acute care SLP completed a complete screening of swallowing, speech, language, and cognition. Findings of the SLP assessment included ZJ's ability to tolerate a speaking valve for awake hours. Mild spastic dysarthria was noted and he was an estimated 80% intelligible at the single word level. A modified barium swallow study was then completed demonstrating severe oropharyngeal dysphagia with aspiration of thin liquids secondary to delayed swallow initiation and silent aspiration. Moderate deficits in attention, short-term memory, and self-awareness, along with severe deficits in inhibition, sequencing, and problem solving were reported. These deficits also impacted language usage at the phrase level and beyond. The SLP initiated a regular diet with nectar thick liquids and ongoing therapy for speech, cognitive-communication, and swallowing. Considerable education was provided to ZJ and his family regarding TBI, his deficits, and next steps in therapy. Based on the SLP evaluation results, along with assessments from other therapy providers, it was determined that inpatient rehabilitation would be the best next level of care for ZJ.

Case 2

BP was a 67-year-old retired professor who was three years post diagnosis of Parkinson's disease. He was experiencing a right-sided tremor, bradykinesia (slowness of movement), and postural instability. He was referred to speech-language pathology services for a speech and swallowing consult. BP stated that people were beginning to have a hard time hearing and understanding him. He also indicated that he had several coughing episodes while eating. Following the interview with BP, his spouse and oldest daughter, the SLP conducted a structure-function evaluation and determined that BP had adequate strength, but scaled down, rapid movements during speech sequences. The SLP also evaluated his respiratory drive using a portable spirometer and established that respiratory capacity appeared within normal limits. Perceptually, the SLP noted reduced loudness, articulatory imprecision, rapid rate of speech, monopitch, and reduced syllable stress—consistent with hypokinetic dysarthria from Parkinson's disease. An objective measure of intelligibility revealed that BP was 94% intelligible when reading sentences, but his intelligibility declined to approximately 85% during conversation (which has an increased cognitive load and lacks the external cuing of the reading task). A modified barium swallow study was completed demonstrating moderate oropharyngeal dysphagia characterized by increased bolus manipulation, oral residuals after the swallow, and delayed swallow initiation resulting in deep penetration with thin liquids. BP was able to increase his loudness when cued, which had a positive effect on his intelligibility. He was subsequently offered

Lee Silverman Voice Treatment, an evidence-based, 4-week, 16-session training program designed to improve loudness and understandability through recalibration of vocal effort and systematic, intensive practice. The SLP also provided compensatory swallowing strategies including alternating liquids and solids along with completing a supraglottic swallow. She discussed communication strategies with BP and his family, such as limiting distractions in the environment during conversations, so that they could maximize the success of their interactions. Given the progressive nature of Parkinson's disease, and the likelihood of worsening speech, swallowing, and possible cognitive abilities, the SLP established a plan following discharge to monitor his level of functioning.

Case 3

J.H. is a 52-year-old male brought to the Emergency Department by his sister due to facial droop, unintelligible speech, and decreased interaction. Upon admission, a CT scan revealed right sided cortical stroke. J.H. has a developmental diagnosis of Down syndrome and lives with his sister and brother-in-law. He spends his days at a day program where he has a job folding papers and stuffing envelopes. SLP was consulted for dysphagia assessment, as J.H. coughed on water during a nursing screener. Upon evaluation, J.H. presented with oral motor features typical of Down syndrome, including low, forward lingual position; tongue thrust swallow with interdental protrusion of the tongue; and low tone. J.H. was able to follow instructions during the exam, though he required a distraction free environment and repetition of simple instructions. He was not oriented to date, though his sister reported that this was typical. J.H. presented with a dysarthria

most like the flaccid type that can be typical of Down syndrome; however, his sister indicated that his volume was decreased and his intelligibility worsened, suggesting a possible UUMN dysarthria from the stroke. A clinical swallow examination revealed a highly disorganized oral phase with anterior loss of material and consistent lingual residue after the swallow. Delayed coughing was noted after the assessment. Although J.H.'s sister reported that he has always had trouble swallowing and is a "messy eater," a modified barium swallow study was completed to further assess the pharyngeal phase of the swallow. Under fluoroscopy, J.H. demonstrated premature spillage of material into the pharynx during bolus manipulation with trace, silent aspiration of liquids before the swallow. He also presented with aspiration during the swallow of thin liquids, which resulted in coughing only when a gross amount of material entered the laryngeal vestibule. Pharyngeal residue was moderate with solids. A puree diet with nectar thick liquids was initiated, and SLP continued to follow for dysphagia management. Soft solid trials were completed in treatment sessions, during which it became evident that J.H. could not control slippery foods, such as canned fruit and pasta. He would swallow whole pieces, resulting in multiple, effortful swallows and delayed coughing. J.H. demonstrated more effective mastication and clearance when presented with crunchy solids, such as goldfish crackers, due to the increased oral-sensory feedback provided. His sister reported success with these textures at home. Education was provided throughout to ensure that J.H.'s sister understood the impact of dysphagia related to stroke superimposed on baseline deficits. J.H. was responsive to cues for increased volume but demonstrated limited carry-over from day to day. Formal cognitive-communication testing was not completed. When J.H. was discharged to a rehabilitation facility, SLP recommendations included continued trials of preferred crunchy solids and providing ongoing family training to ensure safety with PO intake upon discharge home.

Case 4

SB is a 72-year-old woman who was diagnosed with dementia of the Alzheimer's type. She currently resides in an assisted living facility. SB has become increasingly disoriented and agitated. Her son finds it difficult to communicate with her during visits because of her language and memory challenges. The SLP assessed SB's orientation, mental status, episodic memory (through immediate and delayed story retell), spoken/written language comprehension, and language expression. She also screened SB for use of spaced retrieval—an evidence-based therapeutic technique that can help people with declarative memory impairment. The SLP spoke with SB's son to learn more about SB's interests and to request scans of photographs that would be meaningful to SB. The SLP used the pictures to create a memory book. These books are designed to help individuals with dementia to remember relevant information about their history, families, and daily routines in order to maintain orientation/safety, and to provide opportunities for meaningful social communication. The SLP provided instruction to the assisted living facility staff and SB's son regarding the best way to guide a conversation using a memory book. She spoke with them about communication strategies to use when SB was having challenges with word finding, memory, and so for, and the importance of a predictable, daily routine. Finally, the SLP introduced memory aids such as a calendar and daily schedule, and used the spaced retrieval technique to help SB remember to use these aids when she was confused about the date or the schedule. She also labeled several drawers and cabinets in SB's room to help her find items that were important to her.

Case 5

HK is a 63-year-old male patient with a 7-week history of a palpable right neck mass, measuring approximately 3 cm, round and firm. He denied pain to palpation, odynophagia (pain on swallowing), right-sided tinnitus, and otalgia (ear pain). He denied weight loss, fevers, chills, and night sweats. HK was referred to see an ENT by his primary physician and found to have a right base of tongue mass. He had a fine needle biopsy that showed metastatic squamous cell carcinoma. HK completed concurrent chemoradiation for right base of tongue cancer. Due to severe mucositis, a PEG was placed and HK maintained nutrition/hydration via PEG, supplementing with liquids by mouth. He has been cancer free the past 2 years and patient started seeing an SLP to improved swallow function and be weaned off the PEG on an outpatient basis. Per videofluoroscopic swallow study (VFSS), HK exhibited severe oropharyngeal dysphagia characterized by reduced oral bolus control, reduced tongue base retraction, reduced pharyngeal stripping wave, reduced hyolaryngeal excursion and epiglottic inversion, delayed laryngeal vestibule closure, and reduced UES relaxation and opening. Silent aspiration was observed with all consistencies presented. However, the supraglottic swallow (performed twice) did eliminate the aspiration with sips of thin liquid, sips of nectar thick liquid, and puree. Bilateral moderate to severe vallecular and moderate pyriform sinus residue was observed with all consistencies but HK was able to clear it with extra dry swallows and a liquid wash. He completed 12 weeks of weekly swallow treatment, is currently on an advanced diet with thin liquid, and has not been using the PEG for 5 weeks. GI was consulted for PEG removal. A follow-up VFSS revealed mild to moderate oropharyngeal dysphagia characterized by reduced tongue base retraction, reduced pharyngeal stripping wave, reduced hyolaryngeal excursion and epiglottic inversion, delayed laryngeal vestibule closure, and reduced UES relaxation and opening. There was laryngeal penetration and aspiration observed with thin liquid consistency but it was a trace amount and it was spontaneously cleared. The supraglottic swallow eliminated the aspiration with thin liquid. Bilateral mild vallecular and pyriform sinus residue was observed with all consistencies, but the patient was able to clear it with an extra dry swallow. The patient was instructed to continue practicing the swallow exercises at home.

REFERENCES

Abrahams, S., Newton, J., Niven, E., Foley, J., & Bak, T. H. (2014). Screening for cognition and behaviour changes in ALS. *Amyotrohic Lateral Sclerosis and Frontotemporal Degeneration, 15*(1–2), 9–14.

Ajemian, M., Nirmul, G., Anderson, M., Zirlen, D., & Kwasnik, E. (2001). *Archives of Surgery, 136*(4), 434–437.

Aldridge, K. J., & Taylor, N. F. (2012). Dysphagia is a common and serious problem for adults with mental illness: A systematic review. *Dysphagia, 27*, 124–137.

Allain, P., Togher, L., & Azouvi, P. (2018). Social cognition and traumatic brain injury: Current knowledge. *Brain Injury.* https://doi.org/10.1080/02699052.2018.1533143

Allen J., White C. J., Leonard R., & Belafsky P. C. (2010). Effect of cricopharyngeus muscle surgery on the pharynx. *Laryngoscope, 120*, 1498–1503. https://doi.org/10.1002/lary.21002

American Academy of Otolaryngology-Head and Neck Surgery Foundation. (2013). Retrieved from https://www.enthealth.org

American Heart Association (2018). *Classes of Heart Failure.* Retrieved from https://www.heart.org/en/health-topics/heart-failure/what-is-heart-failure/classes-of-heart-failure

American Heart Association/American Stroke Association. (2018a, June 6). *Impact of stroke: Stroke statistics.* Retrieved from https://www.strokeassociation.org/STROKEORG/About-Stroke/Impact-of-Stroke-Stroke-statistics_UCM_310728_Article.jsp

American Heart Association/American Stroke Association. (2018b, August 16). *Learn more stroke warning signs and symptoms.* Retrieved from http://www.strokeassociation.org/STROKEORG/WarningSigns/Learn-More-Stroke-Warning-Signs-and-Symptoms_UCM_451207_Article.jsp#.W_0zVYFKjnF

American Heart Association/American Stroke Association. (2013c, May 23). *Stroke treatments.* Retrieved November 27, 2018, from http://www.strokeassociation.org/STROKEORG/AboutStroke/Stroke-Treatments_UCM_310892_Article.jsp#.W_05bYFKjnE

American Psychiatric Association. (2013). *Diagnostic and statistical manual of mental disorders* (5th ed.). Washington, DC: Author.

American Speech-Language-Hearing Association. (2016). *Scope of practice in speech-language pathology.* Retrieved from http://www.asha.org/policy/

American Speech-Language-Hearing Association. (2017). *ASHA 2017 SLP Health Care Survey: Caseload characteristics.* Available from http://www.asha.org

Arrese, L., & Hutcheson, K. (2018). Framework for speech-language pathology services in patients with oral cavity and oropharyngeal cancers. *Oral and Maxillofacial Surgery Clinics of North America, 30*(4), 397–410.

Asken, B. M., Sullan, M. J., DeKosky, S. T., Jaffee, M. S., & Bauer, R. M. (2017). Research gaps and controversies in chronic traumatic encephalopathy: A review. *JAMA Neurology, 74*(10), 1255–1262.

Aslam, M., & Vaezi, M. (2013). Dysphagia in the elderly. *Gastroenterology Hepatology (N Y), 9*(12), 784–795.

Bajaj, J. (2010). Review article: The modern management of hepatic encephalopathy. *Alimentary Pharmacology & Therapeutics, 31*, 537–547.

Batty, S. (2009). Communication, swallowing and feeding in the intensive care unit patient. *Nursing in Critical Care, 14*(4),175–179.

Bazaz, R., Lee, J., & Yoo, U. (2002). Incidence of dysphagia after anterior cervical spine surgery: A prospective study. *Spine, 22,* 2453–2458.

Beeldman, E., Raaphorst, J., Klein Twennaar, M., de Visser, M., Schmand, B., & de Haanet, R. (2015). The cognitive profile of ALS: A systematic review and meta-analysis update. *Journal of Neurology, Neurosurgery, and Psychiatry.* Advance online publication. https://doi.org/10.1136/jnnp-2015-310734

Belafsky, P. C., Rees, C. J., Allen, J., & Leonard, R. J. (2010). Pharyngeal dilation in cricopharyngeus muscle dysfunction and Zenker diverticulum. *Laryngoscope, 120*(5), 889–894. https://doi.org/10.1002/lary.20874

Belafsky, P. C., & Rees Lintzenich, C. J. (2014). Esophageal phase dysphagia. In R. Leonard & K. A. Kendall, *Dysphagia assessment and treatment planning: A team approach* (3rd ed., pp. 299–308). San Diego, CA: Plural.

Belmont, A., Agar, N., Hugeron, C., Gallais, B., & Azouvi, P. (2006). Fatigue and traumatic brain injury. *Annales de Readaption et de Medecine Physique, 49,* 370–374.

Benigas, J., & Bourgeois, M. (2016). Using spaced Retrieval with external aids to improve use of compensatory strategies during eating for persons with dementia. *American Journal of Speech-Language Pathology, 25,* 321–334.

Beukelman, D., Fager, S., & Nordness, A. (2011). Review article: Communication support for people with ALS. *Neurology Research International, 2011,* 1–6. https://doi.org/10.1155/2011/714693

Bhat, G., Yost, G., & Mahoney, E. (2015). Cognitive function and left ventricular assist device implantation. *Journal of Heart and Lung Transplantation, 34*(11), 1398–1405. https://doi.org/10.1016/j.healun.2015.05.015

Bilney, B., Morris, M., & Perry, A. (2003). Effectiveness of physiotherapy, occupational therapy, and speech pathology for people with Huntington's disease: A systematic review. *Neurorehabilitation and Neural Repair, 17*(1), 12–24.

Binazzi, B., Lanini, B., Romagnoli, I., Garuglieri, S., Stendardi, L., Bianchi, R., . . . Scano, G. (2011). Dyspnea during speech in chronic obstructive pulmonary disease patients: Effects of pulmonary rehabilitation. *Respiration, 81*(5), 379–385. https://doi.org/10.1159/000319553

Boo, H. S., Chik, I., Ngiu, C. S., Lim, S. Y., & Jarmin, R. (2018). High resolution impedance manometry: A necessity or luxury in esophageal motility disorder? *The American Journal of Case Reports, 19,* 998–1003.

Boonstra, A.M., Oosterlaan, J., Sergeant, J.A., & Buitelaar, J.K. (2005). Executive functioning in adult ADHD: A meta-analytic review. *Psychological Medicine, 35*(8), 1097–1108.

Brain Injury Association of America (2018). *Brain injury facts and statistics.* Retrieved from https://www.biausa.org/public-affairs/public-awareness/campaigns/fact-sheet

Bredenoord, A. J., Fox, M., Kahrilas, P. J., Pandolfino, J. E., Schwizer, W., & Smout, A. J.; International High Resolution Manometry Working Group. (2012). Chicago classification criteria of esophageal motility disorders defined in high resolution esophageal pressure topography. *Neurogastroenterology & Motility, 24*(1), 57–65.

Brown J., Chatterjee R., Lowe D., Lewis-Jones H., Rogers S., & Vaughan D. (2005). A new guide to mandibular resection for oral squamous cell carcinoma based on the Cawood and Howell classification of the mandible. *International Journal of Oral and Maxillofacial Surgery, 34,* 834–839.

Brown, R., & Al-Chalabi, A. (2017). Amyotrophic lateral sclerosis. *New England Journal of Medicine, 377*(2), 162–172.

Bülow, M., Olsson, R., & Ekberg, O. (1999). Videomanometric analysis of supraglottic swallow, effortful swallow, and chin tuck in healthy volunteers. *Dysphagia, 14*(2), 67–72.

Castell, J. A., & Castell, D. O. (1997). Recent developments in the manometric assessment of upper esophageal sphincter function and dysfunction. *Digestive Disorders, 15*(Suppl. 1), 28–39. https://doi.org/10.1159/000171619

Centers for Disease Control and Prevention. (2010). *Traumatic brain injury in the United States: Emergency department visits, hospitalizations and deaths 2002–2006.* Retrieved from https://www.cdc.gov/traumaticbraininjury/pdf/blue_book.pdf

Centers for Disease Control and Prevention. (2017, June 27). *Down syndrome data and statistics.* Retrieved from http://www.cdc.gov/ncbddd/birthdefects/downsyndrome/data.html

Chaudhuri, A., & Kennedy, P. (2002). Diagnosis and treatment of viral encephalitis. *Postgraduate Medical Journal, 78,* 575–583.

Cheng, N. T., & Kim, A. S. (2015). Intravenous thrombolysis for acute ischemic stroke within 3 hours versus between 3 and 4.5 hours of symptom onset. *Neurohospitalist, 5*(3), 101–109.

Cherney, L. (2010). Oral reading for language in aphasia: Impact of aphasia severity of cross-modal outcomes in chronic aphasia. *Seminars in Speech and Language, 31*(1), 42–51.

Chiara, T., Martin, A., Davenport, P., & Bolser, D. (2006). Expiratory muscle strength training in persons with multiple sclerosis having mild to moderate disability: Effect on maximal expiratory pressure, pulmonary function, and maximal voluntary cough. *Archives of Physical Medicine and Rehabilitation, 87,* 468–473.

Chieia, M., Oliveira, A., Silva, H., & Gabbai, A. (2010). Amyotrophic lateral sclerosis: Considerations on diagnostic criteria. *Arquivos de Neuro-Psiquiatria, 68*(6), 837–842.

Cicerone, K., Langenbahn, D., Braden, C., Malec, J., Kalmar, K., Fraas, M., . . . Ashman, T. (2011). Evidence-based cognitive rehabilitation: Updated review of the literature from 2003–2008. *Archives of Physical Medicine and Rehabilitation, 92,* 519–530.

Cleveland Clinic. (2018). *Heart failure: Understanding heart failure.* Retrieved from https://my.clevelandclinic.org/health/diseases/17069-heart-failure-understanding-heart-failure

Compton, M. T., Lunden, A., Cleary, S. D., Pauselli, L., Alolayan, Y., Halpern, B., . . . Covington, M. A. (2018). The aprosody of schizophrenia: Computationally derived acoustic phonetic underpinnings of monotone speech. *Schizophrenia Research, 197,* 392–399. https://doi.org/10.1016/j.schres.2018.01.007

Constantinescu, G., Rieger, J., Winget, M., Paulsen, C., & Seikaly, H. (2017). Patient perception of speech outcomes: The relationship between clinical measures and self-perception of speech function following surgical treatment for oral cancer. *American Journal of Speech-Language Pathology, 26,* 241–247.

Cook I. J. (2008). Diagnostic evaluation of dysphagia. *Nature Clinical Practice. Gastroenterology Hepatology, 5,* 393–403.

Cosgrove, J., Alty, J., & Jamieson, S. (2015). Cognitive impairment in Parkinson's disease. *Postgraduate Medical Journal, 91,* 212–220.

Crary, M., Carnaby, G., LaGorio, L., & Carvajal, P. (2012). Functional and physiological outcomes from an exercise-based dysphagia therapy: A pilot investigation of the McNeill Dysphagia Therapy Program. *Archives of Physical Medicine and Rehabilitation, 93,* 1173–1178.

Cumming, T., Marshall, R., & Lazar, R. (2013). Stroke, cognitive deficits, and rehabilitation: Still an incomplete picture. *International Journal of Stroke, 8,* 38–45.

Cvejic, L., & Bardin, P. G. (2018). Swallow and aspiration in chronic obstructive pulmonary disease. *American Journal of Respiratory and Critical Care Medicine, 198*(9), 1122–1129.

Darley, F., Brown, J., & Goldstein, N. (1972). Dysarthria in multiple sclerosis. *Journal of Speech, Language, and Hearing Research, 15,* 229–245.

De Swart, B., van Engelen, B., van de Kerkhof, J., & Maassen, B. (2004). Myotonia and flaccid dysarthria in patients with adult onset myotonic dystrophy. *Journal of Neurology, Neurosurgery, and Psychiatry, 75,* 1480–1482.

Dewan, M. C., Rattani, A., Gupta, S., Baticulon, R. E., Hung, Y. C., Punchak, M., . . . Park, K. B. (2018). Estimating the global incidence of traumatic brain injury. *Journal of Neurosurgery, 27,* 1–18.

Dietrich-Burns, K., Lewis, B., Lesley, D., & Solomon, N. P. (2013). Dysphagia in a case of Bickerstaff Brainstem Encephalitis. *Military Medicine, 178*(1), e121–e124.

Ding, H., Duan, Z., Yang, D., Zhang, Z., Wang, L., Sun, X., . . . Chen, J. D. Z. (2017). High-resolution manometry in patients with and without globus pharyngeus and/or symptoms of laryngopharyngeal reflux. *BMC Gastroenterology, 17*(1), 109. https://doi.org/10.1186/s12876-017-0666-x

Dolce, G., Arcuri, F., Carozzo, S., Cortese, M., Greco, P., Lucca, L., & Riganello, F. (2015). Care and neurorehabilitation in the disorder of consciousness: A model in progress. *Scientific World Journal, 2015*, 463829.

Duffy, J. R. (2013). *Motor speech disorders* (3rd ed.). St. Louis, MO: Elsevier Mosby.

Dwivedi, R. C., St. Rose, S., Chisholm, E. J., Bisase, B., Amen F., Nutting, C. M., . . . Kazi R. (2012). Evaluation of speech outcomes using English version of the Speech Handicap Index in a cohort of head and neck cancer patients. *Oral Oncology, 48*(6), 547–553.

Dzioba, A., Aalto, D., Papadopoulos-Nydam, G., Seikaly, H., Rieger, J., Wolfaardt, J., . . . Laine, J.; Head and Neck Research Network. (2017). Functional and quality of life outcomes after partial glossectomy: A multi-institutional longitudinal study of the head and neck research network. *Journal of Otolaryngology-Head & Neck Surgery, 46*(1), 56.

Edmonds, L. (2016). A review of verb network strengthening treatment: Theory, methods, results, and clinical implications. *Top Language Disorders, 36*(2), 123–135.

Efstratiadou, E., Papathanasiou, I., Holland, R., Archonti, A., & Hilari, K. (2018). A systematic review of semantic feature analysis therapy studies for aphasia. *Journal of Speech, Language, and Hearing Research, 61*, 1261–1278.

Ekberg, O., & Wahlgren, L. (1985). Pharyngeal dysfunctions and their interrelationship in patients with dysphagia. *Acta Radiologica: Diagnosis (Stockh), 26*(6), 659–664.

Emery, A. (2002). The muscular dystrophies. *Lancet, 359*(9307), 687–695.

Esbensen, A. (2010). Health conditions associated with aging and end of life of adults with Down syndrome. *International Review of Research in Mental Retardation, 39*(C), 107–126.

European Delirium Association and American Delirium Society. (2014). The DSM-5 criteria, level of arousal and delirium diagnosis: Inclusiveness is safer. *BMC Medicine, 12*, 141.

Exner, N., Lutz, N., Haass, C., & Winklhofer, K. (2012). Mitochondrial dysfunction in Parkinson's disease: Molecular mechanisms and pathophysiological consequences. *The EMBO Journal, 31*(14), 3038–3062.

Farmer, C., Krull, H., Concannon, T., Simmons, M., Pillemer, F., Ruder, T., & Hepner, K. (2017). Understanding treatment of mild traumatic brain injury in the military health system. *Rand Health Quarterly, 6*(2), 11.

Faul, M., Xu, L., Wald, M., & Coronado, V. (2010). *Traumatic brain injury in the United States: Emergency department visits, hospitalizations, and deaths.* Atlanta, GA: Centers for Disease Control and Prevention, National Center for Injury Prevention and Control. Retrieved from https://stacks.cdc.gov/view/cdc/5571

Felmingham, K., Baguley, I., & Green, A. (2004). Effects of diffuse axonal injury on speed of information processing following severe traumatic brain injury. *Neuropsychology, 18*(3), 564–571.

Fennell, E., & Dikel, T. (2001). Cognitive and neuropsychological functioning in children with cerebral palsy. *Journal of Child Neurology, 16*(1), 58–63.

Flowers, H., Skoretz, S., Streiner, D., Silver, F., & Martino, R. (2011). MRI-Based neuroanatomical predictors ofd after acute ischemic stroke: A systematic review and meta-analysis. *Cerebrovascular Diseases, 32*, 1–10.

Flynn, A., Macaluso, M., D'Empaire, I., & Troutman, M. (2015). Wernicke's encephalopathy: Increasing clinician awareness of this serious, enigmatic, yet treatable disease. *Primary Care Companion for CNS Disorders, 17*(3). https://doi.org/10.4088/PCC.14r01738

Frank, S. (2014). Treatment of Huntington's disease. *Neurotherapeutics, 11*, 153–160.

Franke, B., Michelini, G., Asherson, P., Banaschewski, T., Bilbow, A., Buitelaar, J. K., . . . Reif, A. (2018). Live fast, die young? A review on the developmental trajectories of ADHD across the lifespan. *European Neuropsychopharmacology, 28*(10), 1059–1088. https://doi.org/10.1016/j.euroneuro.2018.08.001

Frempong-Boadu, A., Houten, K., Osborn, B., Opulencia, J., Kells, L., Guida, D. D., & Le Roux, P. D. (2002). Swallowing and speech dysfunction in patients undergoing anterior cervical discectomy and fusion: A prospective, objective preoperative and postoperative assessment. *Journal of Spinal Disorders and Techniques, 5*, 362–368.

Fried-Oken, M., Mooney, A., & Peters, B. (2015). Supporting communication for patients with neurodegenerative disease. *NeuroRehabilitation, 37*, 69–87.

Fuermaier, A. B. M., Tucha, L., Koerts, J., Aschenbrenner, S., Weisbrod, M., Lange, K. W., & Tucha, O. (2014). Cognitive complaints of adults with attention deficit hyperactivity disorder. *Clinical Neuropsychologist, 28*(7), 1104–1122. https://doi.org/10.1080/13854046.2014.964325

Fuermaier, A. B. M., Tucha, L., Koerts, J., Hauser, J., Kaunzinger, I., Aschenbrenner, S., . . . Tucha, O. (2015). Cognitive impairment in adult ADHD-perspective matters. *Neuropsychology, 29*(1), 45–58. https://doi.org/10.1037/neu0000108

Gage, B. F., Waterman, A. D., Shannon, W., Boechler, M., Rich, M. W., & Radford, M. J. (2001). Validation of clinical classification schemes for predicting stroke: Results from the National Registry of Atrial Fibrillation. *JAMA, 285*(22), 2864–2870.

Gerber, S., Gengler, C., Gratz, K. W., & Kruse, A. L. (2011). The impact of frozen sections on final surgical margins in squamous cell carcinoma of the oral cavity and lips: A retrospective analysis over an 11 years period. *Head & Neck Oncology, 3,* 56.

Ghajar, J. (2000). Traumatic brain injury. *Lancet, 356*(9233), 923–929.

Giacino, J., Kalmar, K., & Whyte, J. (2004). The JFK Coma Recovery Scale-Revised: Measurement characteristics and diagnostic utility. *Archives of Physical Medicine and Rehabilitation, 85*(12), 2020–2029.

Giusti, A., & Giambuzzi, M. (2008). Management of dysphagia in patients affected by multiple sclerosis: State of the art. *Neurological Sciences, 29*(s4), 364–366.

Goetz, C. G., Fahn, S., Martinez-Martin, P., Poewe, W., Sampaio, C., Stebbins, G. T., . . . Lapelle, N. (2007). Movement disorder society-sponsored revision of the Unified Parkinson's Disease Rating Scale (MDS-UPDRS): Process, format, and clinimetric testing plan. *Movement Disorders, 22*(1), 41–47.

Golper, L. A. C., Klaben, B. K., & Miller, C. K. (2019). *Medical speech-language pathology: A desk reference* (4th ed.). San Diego, CA: Plural.

Gooch, C. L., Pracht, E., & Borenstein, A. R. (2017). The burden of neurological disease in the United States: A summary report and call to action. *Annals of Neurology, 81*(4), 479–484.

Goodglass, H., Kaplan, E., & Baressi, B. (2000). *The assessment of aphasia and related disorders* (3rd ed.). Boston, MA: Lippincott, Williams, & Wilkins.

Graff-Radford, J., Jones, D. T., Strand, E. A., Rabinstein, A. A., Duffy, J. R., & Josephs, K. A. (2014). The neuroanatomy of pure apraxia of speech in stroke. *Brain and Language, 129,* 43–46.

Granell, J., Garrido, L., Millas, T., & Gutierrez-Fonseca, R. (2012). Management of oropharyngeal dysphagia in laryngeal and hypopharyngeal cancer. *International Journal of Otolaryngology,* 1–9.

Groher, M., & Crary, M. (2010). *Dysphagia: Clinical management in adults and children* (p. 108). Maryland Heights, MO: Mosby Elsevier.

Gurkin, S., Parikshak, M., Kralovich, K., Horst, H., Agarwal, V., & Payne, N. (2002) Indicators for tracheostomy in patients with traumatic brain injury. *American Surgery, 88*(4), 324–328.

Gyawali C. P., Bredenoord A. J., Conklin J. L., Fox, M., Pandolfino, J. E., Peters, J. H., . . . Vaezi, M. F. (2013). Evaluation of esophageal motor function in clinical practice. *Neurogastroenterology Motility, 25*(2), 99–133. https://doi.org/10.1111/nmo.12071

Haak, P., Lenski, M., Hidecker, M., Li, M., & Paneth, N. (2009). Cerebral palsy and aging. *Developmental Medicine & Child Neurology, 51*(Suppl. 4), 16–23.

Hadjikoutis, S., & Wiles, C. (2001). Respiratory complications related to bulbar dysfunction in motor neuron disease. *Acta Neurologica Scandinavia, 103,* 207–213.

Hagen, C. (2000, February). *Rancho levels of cognitive functioning–Revised.* Paper presented at TBI Rehabilitation in a Managed Care Environment: An Interdisciplinary Approach to Rehabilitation, Continuing Education Programs of America, San Antonio, Texas.

Haller, M., Iwanik, M., & Shen, H. (2011). Clinically relevant anatomy of high anterior cervical approach. *Spine, 25,* 2116–2121.

Hamadani, M., & Awan, F. (2006). Role of thiamine in managing ifosfamide-induced encephalopathy. *Journal of Oncology Pharmacy Practice, 12*, 237–239.

Hamdy, S., Mikulis, D. J., Crawley, A., Xue, S., Lau, H., Henry, S., & Diamant, N. E. (1999). Cortical activation during human volitional swallowing: An event-related fMRI study. *American Journal of Physiology, 277*(1), G219–G225.

Hansen, K., Chenoweth, M., Thompson, H., & Strouss, A. (2018). Role of the speech-language pathologist (SLP) in the head and neck cancer team. *Cancer Treatment and Research, 174*, 31–42. https://doi.org/10.1007/978-3-319-65421-8_3

Hartelius, L., Theodoros, D., Cahill, L., & Lilivik, M. (2003). Comparability of perceptual analysis of speech characteristics in Australian and Swedish speakers with multiple sclerosis. *Folia Phoniatrica et Logopaedica, 55*, 177–188.

Harvard NeuroDiscovery Center. (n.d.). *The challenge of neurodegenerative diseases.* Retrieved from https://neurodiscovery.harvard.edu/challenge

Hashem, M., Nelliot, A., & Needham, D. (2016). Early mobilization and rehabilitation in the ICU: Moving back to the future. *Respiratory Care Journal, 61*(7), 971–979. https://doi.org/10.4187/respcare.04741

Hatlebakk, J., Castell, J., Spiegel, J., Paoletti, V., Katz, P., & Castell, D. (1998). Dilatation therapy for dysphagia in patients with upper esophageal sphincter dysfunction—manometric and symptomatic response. *Diseases of the Esophagus, 11*(4).

Heegaard, W., & Biros, M. (2007). Traumatic brain injury. *Emergency Medicine Clinics of North America, 25*, 655–678.

Heemskerk, A. & Roos, R. (2012). Aspiration pneumonia and death in Huntington's disease. *PLoS Currents, 30*(4), RRN1293.

Helland, W. A., Helland, T., & Heimann, M. (2014). Language profiles and mental health problems in children with specific language impairment and children with ADHD. *Journal of Attention Disorders, 18*(3), 226–235. https://doi.org/10.1177/1087054712441705

Herridge, M. S., Tansey, C. M., Matté, A., Tomlinson, G., Diaz-Granados, N., Cooper, A., . . . Cheung, A. M. (2011). Functional disability 5 years after acute respiratory distress syndrome. *New England Journal of Medicine, 364*(14), 1293–1304. https://doi.org/10.1056/NEJMoa1011802

Hila, A., Castell, J., & Castell, D. (2001). Pharyngeal and upper esophageal sphincter manometry in the evaluation of dysphagia. *Journal of Clinical Gastroenterology, 33*(5), 355–361.

Hillis, A. (2007). Aphasia: Progress in the last quarter of a century. *Neurology, 69*, 200–213.

Hirano, I., & Kahrilas, J. (2012). Dysphagia. *Harrison's principles of internal medicine* (18th ed.). New York, NY: McGraw-Hill,

Hoehn, M.M., & Yahr, M. D. (1967). Parkinsonism: Onset, progression, and mortality. *Neurology, 17*, 427–442.

Hopper, T., Bourgeois, M., Pimentel, J., Qualls, C., Hickey, E., Frymark, T., & Schooling, T. (2013). An evidence-based systematic review on cognitive interventions for individuals with dementia. *American Journal of Speech-Language Pathology, 22*, 126–145.

Husa, A. P., Moilanen, J., Murray, G. K., Marttila, R., Haapea, M., Rannikko, I., . . . Jääskeläinen, E. (2017). Lifetime antipsychotic medication and cognitive performance in schizophrenia at age 43 years in a general population birth cohort. *Psychiatry Research, 247*, 130–138. https://doi.org/10.17863/CAM.7551

Iacobone, E., Bailly-Salin, J., Polito, A., Friedman, D., Stevens, R., & Sharshar, T. (2009). Sepsis-associated encephalopathy and its differential diagnosis. *Critical Care Medicine, 37*(1), S331–S336.

Jackson, A., Maybee, J., Moran, M., Wolter-Warmerdam, K., & Hickey, F. (2016). Clinical characteristics of dysphagia in children with Down syndrome. *Dysphagia, 31*(5), 663–671.

Jacobi, I., van der Molen, L., Huiskens, H., van Rossum, M. A., & Hilgers, F. J. (2010). Voice and speech outcomes of chemoradiation for advanced head and neck cancer: A systematic review. *European Archives of Oto-Rhino-Laryngology, 267*(10), 1495–1505.

Jacobs, B., Drew, R., Ogletree, B., & Pierce, K. (2004). Augmentative and alternative communication (AAC) for adults with severe aphasia: where we stand and how we can go further.

Disability and Rehabilitation, 26(21–22), 1231–1240.

Jankovic, J. (2008). Parkinson's disease: Clinical features and diagnosis. *Journal of Neurology, Neurosurgery, and Psychiatry, 79,* 368–376.

Jennings, K., Siroky, D., & Jackson, C. (1992). Swallowing problems after excision of tumors of the skull base: Diagnosis and management in 12 patients. *Dysphagia, 7,* 40–44.

Johnston, B. T. (2017). Esophageal dysphagia: A stepwise approach to diagnosis and management. *Lancet Gastroenterology Hepatology, 2,* 604–609.

Johnson, K. L., Speirs, L., Mitchell, A., Przybyl, H., Anderson, D., Manos, B., . . . Winchester, K. (2018). Validation of a postextubation dysphagia screening tool for patients after prolonged endotracheal intubation. *American Journal of Critical Care, 27*(2), 89–96.

Jones, D., Aloraini, A., Gowing, S., & Cools-Lartigue, J. (2016). Evolving management of Zenker's diverticulum in endoscopic era: A North American experience. *World Journal of Surgery, 40*(6), 1390–1396.

Joyal, M., Bonneau, A., & Fecteau, S. (2016). Speech and language therapies to improve pragmatics and discourse skills in patients with schizophrenia. *Psychiatry Research, 240,* 88–95.

Kagel, M., & Leopold, N. (1992). Dysphagia in Huntington's disease: A 16-year retrospective. *Dysphagia, 7,* 106–114.

Kalabalik, J., Brunetti, L., & El-Srougy, R. (2014). Intensive care unit delirium: A review of the literature. *Journal of Pharmacy Practice, 27*(2), 195–207. https://doi.org/10.1177/08971900 13513804

Kalf, J. G., de Swart, B. J., Bloem, B. R., & Munnecke, M. (2012). Prevalence of oropharyngeal dysphagia in Parkinson's disease: A meta-analysis. *Parkinsonism and Related Disorders, 18,* 311–315.

Kalish, V. B., Gillham, J. E., & Unwin, B. K. (2014). Delirium in older persons: Evaluation and management. *American Family Physician, 90*(3), 150–158.

Kennedy, M., & Coelho, C. (2005). Self-regulation after traumatic brain injury: A framework for intervention of memory and problem solving. *Seminars in Speech and Language, 26*(4), 242–255.

Kent, R. D., & Vorperien, H. K. (2013). Speech impairment in Down syndrome: A review. *Journal of Speech, Language, and Hearing Research, 56*(1), 178–210.

Kepler, K., Rihn, J. A., Bennett, J. D., Anderson, D. G., Vaccaro, A. R., Albert, T. J., & Hilibrand, A. S. (2012). Dysphagia and soft-tissue swelling after anterior cervical surgery: A radiographic analysis. *The Spine Journal, 12*(8), 639–644.

Kerawala, C., Roques, T., Jeannon, J. P., & Bisase, B. (2016). Oral cavity and lip cancer: United Kingdom National Multidisciplinary Guidelines. *Journal of Laryngology and Otology, 130*(S2), S83–S89.

Khariwala, S., Vivek, P., Lorenz, R., Esclamado, M., Wood, B., Strome, M., & Alam, S. (2007). Swallowing outcomes after microvascular head and neck reconstruction: A prospective review of 191 cases. *Laryngoscope, 117*(8), 1359–1363.

Kim, Y., & Kim, J. (2012). Toxic encephalopathy. *Safety and Health at Work, 3,* 243–256.

Körner, S., Siniawski, M., Kollewe, K., Rath, K., Krampel, K., Zapf, A., & Petri, S. (2013). Speech therapy and communication device: Impact on quality of life and mood in patients with amyotrophic lateral sclerosis. *Amyotrophic Lateral Sclerosis and Frontotemporal Degeneration, 14,* 20–25.

Korrel, H., Mueller, K. L., Silk, T., Anderson, V., & Sciberras, E. (2017). Research review: Language problems in children with attention-deficit hyperactivity disorder—a systematic meta-analytic review. *Journal of Child Psychology and Psychiatry, 58*(6), 640–654. https://doi.org/10.1111/jcpp.12688

Kotz, T., Federman, D., Kao, J., Milman, L., Packer, S., Lopez-Prieto, C., . . . Genden, E. M. (2012). Prophylactic swallowing exercises in patients with head and neck cancer undergoing chemoradiation: A randomized trial. *Archives of Otolaryngology-Head & Neck Surgery, 138,* 376–382.

Koufman, J. A., Aviv, J. E., Casiano, R. R., & Shaw, G. Y. (2002). Laryngopharyngeal reflux, position statement of the Committee of Speech, Voice, and Swallowing Disorders of the American Academy of Otolaryngology-Head and Neck Surgery. *Otolaryngology-Head and Neck Surgery, 127*, 32–35.

Kuhn M., & Belafsky P. (2013). Management of cricopharyngeus muscle dysfunction. *Otolaryngologic Clinics of North America, 46*, 1087–1099.

Kulkarni, D., Kamath, V., & Stewart, J. (2017). Swallowing disorders in schizophrenia. *Dysphagia, 32*(4), 467–471. https://doi.org/10.1007/s00455–017–9802–6

Kumar, C., Salzman, B., & Colburn, J. L. (2018). Preoperative assessment in older adults: A comprehensive approach. *American Family Physician, 98*(4), 214–220.

Lee, J., Bazaz, R., Furey, G., & Yoo, J. (2007). Risk factors for dysphagia after anterior cervical spine surgery: A two-year prospective cohort study. *The Spine Journal, 7*, 141–147.

Lee, W., Yeom, J., Lee, W., Seo, H., Oh, B., & Han, T. (2016). Characteristics of dysphagia in severe traumatic brain injury patients: A comparison with stroke patients. *Annals of Rehabilitation Medicine, 40*(3), 432–439.

Lee, Y., Lim, M. R., & Albert, T. J. (2011). Dysphagia after anterior cervical spine surgery: Pathophysiology, incidence, and prevention. *Spine, 36*, 2286–2292.

Leonard, R., & Belafsky, P. (2011). Dysphagia following cervical spine surgery with anterior instrumentation: Evidence from fluoroscopic swallow studies. *Spine, 25*, 2217–2223.

Leonard, R., & Kendall, K. (2014). *Dysphagia assessment and treatment planning: A team approach* (3rd ed.). San Diego, CA: Plural.

Leto, L., & Feola, M. (2014). Cognitive impairment in heart failure patients. *Journal of Geriatric Cardiology, 11*(4), 316–328. https://doi.org/10.11909/j.issn.1671–5411.2014.04.007

Levin, H., O'Donnell, V., & Grossman, R. (1979). The Galveston Orientation and Amnesia Test: A practical scale to assess cognition after head injury. *Journal of Nervous and Mental Diseases, 167*(11), 675–684.

Lewin, J., Teng, S., & Kotz, T. (2016). Speech and swallowing rehabilitation of the patient with head and neck cancer. *UpToDate, Inc.* (1). Retrieved from http://www.uptodate.com/contents/speech-and-swallowing-rehabilita tion-of-the-patient-with-head-and-neck-cancer#H1

Li, A. W. Y., Viñas-Guasch, N., Hui, C. L. M., Chang, W-C., Chan, S. K. W., Lee, E. H. M., & Chen, E. Y. H. (2017). Verbal working memory in schizophrenia: The role of syntax in facilitating serial recall. *Schizophrenia Research, 192*, 294–299. https://doi.org/10.1016/j.schres.2017.04.008

Lindsey, A., Hurley, E., Mozeiko, J., & Coelho, C. (2018). Follow-up on the Story Goodness Index for characterizing discourse deficits following traumatic brain injury. *American Journal of Speech Language Pathology*, 1–11. https://doi.org/10.1044/2018_AJSLP-17-0151

Litvan, I., Goldman, J., Tröster, A., Schmand, B., Weintraub, D., Petersen, R., & Emre, M. (2012). Diagnostic criteria for mild cognitive impairment in Parkinson's disease: Movement disorder society task force guidelines. *Movement Disorders, 27*(3), 349–356.

Logemann, J. A., Pauloski, B. R., Rademaker, A. W., & Colangelo, L. A. (1997) Speech and swallowing rehabilitation for head and neck cancer patients. *Oncology, 11*, 651–659.

Lovera, J., & Kovner, B. (2012). Cognitive impairment in multiple sclerosis. *Current Neurology and Neuroscience Reports, 12*(5), 618–627.

Lynch, Y. T., Clark, B. J., Macht, M., White, S. D., Taylor, H., Wimbish, T., & Moss, M. (2017). The accuracy of the bedside swallowing evaluation for detecting aspiration in survivors of acute respiratory failure. *Journal of Critical Care, 39*, 143–148. https://doi.org/10.1016/j.jcrc.2017.02.013

Mackay, L., Morgan, A., & Bernstein, B. (1999). Swallowing disorders in severe brain injury: Risk factors affecting return to oral intake. *Archives of Physical Medicine and Rehabilitation, 80*, 365–371.

Mackenzie, C. (2011). Dysarthria in stroke: A narrative review of its description and the outcome of intervention. *International Journal of Speech-Language Pathology, 13*(2), 125–136.

Malandraki, G., Rajappa, A., Kantarcigil, C., Wagner, E., Ivey, C., & Youse, K. (2016). The intensive dysphagia rehabilitation approach applied to patients with neurogenic dysphagia: A case series design study. *Archives of Physical Medicine and Rehabilitation, 97,* 567–574.

Mann, G., Hankey, G., & Cameron, D. (2000). Swallowing disorders following acute stroke: Prevalence and diagnostic accuracy. *Cerebrovascular Diseases, 10,* 380–386.

Martin, E., Neary, A., & Diamant, E. (1997). Dysphagia following anterior cervical spine surgery. *Dysphagia, 1,* 2–8.

Martino, R., Foley, N., Bhogal, S., Diamant, N., Speechley, M., & Teasell, R. (2005). Dysphagia after stroke: Incidence, diagnosis, and pulmonary complications. *Stroke, 36,* 2756–2763.

McConnel, F. M., Logemann, J. A., Rademaker, A. W., Pauloski, B. R., Baker, S. R., Lewin, J., . . . Baker, T. (1994), Surgical variables affecting postoperative swallowing efficiency in oral cancer patients: A pilot study. *Laryngoscope, 104,* 87–90.

McDonald, I., Compston, A., Edan, G., Goodkin, D., Hartung, H., Lublin, F., & Wolinsky, J. S. (2001). Recommended diagnostic criteria for multiple sclerosis: Guidelines from the International Panel on the Diagnosis of Multiple Sclerosis. *Annals of Neurology, 50,* 121–127.

McKee, A. C., Cairns, N. J., Dickson, D. W., Folkerth, R. D., Keene, C. D., Litvan, I., . . . Gordon, W. A. (2016). The first NINDS/NIBIB consensus meeting to define neuropathological criteria for the diagnosis of chronic traumatic encephalopathy. *Acta Neuropathologica, 13*(1), 75–86.

McKee, A., Cantu, R., Nowinski, C., Hedley-Whyte, T., Gavett, B., Budson, A . . . Stern, R. (2009). Chronic traumatic encephalopathy in athletes: Progressive taupathy after repetitive head injury. *Journal of Neuropathology and Experimental Neurology, 68*(7), 709–735.

McKhanna, G., Knopmanc, D., Chertkowd, H., Hymanf, B., Jack, C., Kawas, C. H . . . Phelps, C. H. (2011). The diagnosis of dementia due to Alzheimer's disease: Recommendations from the National Institute on Aging-Alzheimer's Association workgroups on diagnostic guidelines for Alzheimer's disease. *Alzheimer's & Dementia, 7,* 263–269.

Menezes, E., Santos, F., & Alves, F. (2017). Cerebral palsy dysphagia: A systematic review. *Revista Cefac Speech, Language, Hearing Sciences Education Journal, 19*(4), 565–573.

Mercuri, E., & Muntoni, F. (2013). Muscular dystrophies. *Lancet, 381,* 845–860.

Michou, E., Baijens, L., Rofes, L., Cartgena, P. S., & Clavé, P. (2013). Oropharyngeal swallowing disorders in Parkinson's disease: Revisited. *International Journal of Speech and Language Pathology and Audiology, 1,* 76–88.

Miller, D., & Leary, S. (2007). Primary-progressive multiple sclerosis. *Lancet Neurology, 6,* 903–912.

Miranda, A., Mercader, J., Fernández, M., & Colomer, C. (2017). Reading performance of young adults with ADHD diagnosed in childhood. *Journal of Attention Disorders, 21*(4), 294–304.

Mitchell, C., Bowen, A., Tyson, S., Butterfint, Z., & Conroy, P. (2017). Interventions for dysarthria due to stroke and other adult-acquired, non-progressive brain injury. *Cochrane Database Systematic Reviews,* https://doi.org/10.1002/14651858.CD002088.pub3

Montoya, A., Price, B., Menear, M., & Lepage, M. (2006). Brain imaging and cognitive dysfunctions in Huntington's disease. *Journal of Psychiatry and Neuroscience, 31*(1), 21–29.

Moraes, D., Sassi, F., Mangilli, L., Zilberstein, B., & de Andrade, C. (2013). Clinical prognostic indicators of dysphagia following prolonged orotracheal intubation in ICU patients. *Critical Care, 17,* R243.

Morgan, L. (2017). Exercise-based dysphagia rehabilitation: Past, present, and future. *Perspectives of the ASHA Special Interest Groups* (SIG 13), *2*(1), 36–43.

Mozaffarian, D., Benjamin, E. J., Go, A. S., Arnett, D. K., Blaha, M.J., Cushman, M., . . . Turner, M. (2016). Heart disease and stroke statistics—2016 update: A report from the American Heart Association. *Circulation, 133,* e38–e360. https://doi.org/10.1161/CIR.0000000000000350

Muench, J. & Hamer, A. M. (2010). Adverse effects of antipsychotic medications. *American Family Physician, 81*(5), 617–622. Retrieved from https://www.clinicalkey.es/playcontent/1-s2.0-S0002838X10601104

Mulloy, A., Lang, R., O'Reilly, M., Sigafoos, J., Lancioni, G., & Rispoli, M. (2009).

Gluten-free and casein-free diets in the treatment of autism spectrum disorders: A systematic review. *Research in Autism Spectrum Disorders.* https://doi.org/10.1016/j.rasd.2009.10.008

Muralidharan, A., Finch, A., Bowie, C. R., & Harvey, P. D. (2018). Thought, language, and communication deficits and association with everyday functional outcomes among community-dwelling middle-aged and older adults with schizophrenia. *Schizophrenia Research, 196,* 29–34. https://doi.org/10.1016/j.schres.2017.07.017

Namaki, S., Tanaka, T., Hara, Y., Ohki, H., Shinohara, M., & Yonehara, Y. (2011). Videofluorographic evaluation of dysphagia before and after modification of the flap and scar in patients with oral cancer, *Journal of Plastic Surgery and Hand Surgery, 45*(3), 136–142.

National Alliance on Mental Illness (2018). *ADHD.* Retrieved from https://www.nami.org/

National Heart, Lung, and Blood Institute. (2018). *Heart failure.* Retrieved from https://www.nhlbi.nih.gov/health-topics/heart-failure

National Institute of Environmental Health Sciences (NIH). (2018, August 6). *Neurodegenerative diseases.* Retrieved from https://www.niehs.nih.gov/research/supported/health/neurodegenerative/index.cfm

National Institute of Health. (n.d.). *NIH fact sheet: Multiple sclerosis.* Retrieved from https://report.nih.gov/nihfactsheets/ViewFactSheet.aspx?csid=103

National Institute of Neurological Disorders and Stroke. (2018a, June 12). *Encephalopathy information page.* Retrieved from https://www.ninds.nih.gov/Disorders/All-Disorders/Encephalopathy-Information-Page

National Institute of Neurological Disorders and Stroke. (2018, July 16). *Meningitis and encephalitis fact sheet.* Retrieved from https://www.ninds.nih.gov/Disorders/Patient-Caregiver-Education/Fact-Sheets/Meningitis-and-Encephalitis-Fact-Sheet

National Institute of Neurological Disorders and Stroke. (2018b, July 6). *Neurological complications of AIDS fact sheet.* Retrieved from https://www.ninds.nih.gov/Disorders/Patient-Caregiver-Education/Fact-Sheets/Neurological-Complications-AIDS-Fact-Sheet

Naunheim, M., R., & Carroll, T. L. (2017). Benign vocal fold lesions: update on nomenclature, cause, diagnosis, and treatment. *Current Opinion in Otolaryngology & Head and Neck Surgery, 25*(6), 453–458.

Nazem, S., Siderowf, A., Duda, J., Have, T., Colcher, A., Horn, S., . . . Weintraub, D. (2009). Montreal Cognitive Assessment performance in patients with Parkinson's disease with "Normal" global cognition according to Mini-Mental State Examination Score. *Journal of the American Geriatrics Society, 57*(2), 304–308.

Needham, D. M. (2008). Mobilizing patients in the intensive care unit. *JAMA, 300*(14), 1685. https://doi.org/10.1001/jama.300.14.1685

Neurodegenerative diseases. (2018, August 6). Retrieved from https://www.niehs.nih.gov/research/supported/health/neurodegenerative/index.cfm

Nixon, D. (2018). Down syndrome, obesity, Alzheimer's disease, and cancer: A brief review and hypothesis. *Brain Sciences, 8*(4), 53.

Novack, T. (2000). *The orientation log.* The Center for Outcome Measures in Brain Injury. Retrieved from http://www.tbims.org/combi/olog

Nys, G., van Zandvoort, M., Kort, P., Jansen, B., de Haan, E., & Kapelle, L. (2007). Cognitive disorders in acute stroke: Prevalence and clinical determinants. *Cerebrovascular Disorders, 23,* 408–416.

O'Brien, K., & Kennedy, M. (2018). Predicting remembering: Judgments of prospective memory after traumatic brain injury. *Journal of Speech, Language, and Hearing Research, 61,* 1393–1408.

Oelsner, E. C., Loehr, L. R., Henderson, A. G., Donohue, K. M., Enright, P. L., Kalhan, R., . . . Barr, R. G. (2016). Classifying chronic lower respiratory disease events in epidemiologic cohort studies. *Annals of the American Thoracic Society, 13*(7), 1057–1066. https://doi.org/10.1513/AnnalsATS.201601–063OC

Olsson, R., Castell, J., Johnston, B., Ekberg, O., & Castell, D. (1997). Combined videomanometric identification of abnormalities related to pharyngeal retention. *Acta Radiologica, 39*(4), 405–409

Olsson, R., & Ekberg, O. (1995). Videomanometry of the pharynx in dysphagic patients with a posterior cricopharyngeal indentation. *Acta Radiologica, 2,* 597–601.

Olsson, R., Nilsson, H., & Ekberg, O. (1994). Simultaneous videoradiography and computerized pharyngeal manometry-videomanometry. *Acta Radiologica, 35,* (1).

Oren, S., Willerton, C., & Small, J. (2014). Effects of spaced retrieval training on semantic memory in Alzheimer's disease: A systematic review. *Journal of Speech, Language, and Hearing Research, 57,* 247–270.

O'Walker, F. (2007). Huntington's disease. *Lancet, 369,* 218–228.

Pandharipande, P. P., Girard, T. D., Jackson, J. C., Morandi, A., Thompson, J. L., Pun, B. T., . . . Ely, E. W. (2013). Long-term cognitive impairment after critical illness. *New England Journal of Medicine, 369*(14), 1306–1316. https://doi .org/10.1056/NEJMoa1301372

Pape, T., Heinemann, A., Kelly, J., Hurder, A., & Lundgren, S. (2005). A measure of neurobehavioral functioning after coma. Part I: Theory, reliability, and validity of the Disorders of Consciousness Scale. *Journal of Rehabilitation Research and Development, 42*(1), 1–18.

Pape, T., Rosenow, J., Steiner, M., Parrish, T., Guernon, A., Harton, B., & Nemeth, A. (2015). Placebo-controlled trial of familiar auditory sensory training for acute severe traumatic brain injury: A preliminary report. *Neurorehabilitation and Neural Repair, 29*(6), 537–547.

Patel R. S., Goldstein D. P., Brown D., Irish, J., Gullane, P. J., & Gilbert, R. W. (2010) Circumferential pharyngeal reconstruction: History, critical analysis of techniques, and current therapeutic recommendations. *Head & Neck, 32,* 109–120.

Patti, F. (2009). Cognitive impairment in multiple sclerosis. *Multiple Sclerosis Journal, 15*(1), 2–8.

Paul, D. (2013). A quick guide to DSM-V. *The ASHA Leader, 18,* 52–54. Retrieved from http://leader.pubs.asha.org/article.aspx?article id=1785031

Paul, R., & Norbury, C. (2012). *Language disorders from infancy through adolescence: Listening,* speaking, reading, writing, and communicating (4th ed.). St. Louis, MO: Elsevier Mosby.

Pauloski, B. R., Rademaker, A. W., Lazarus, C., Boeckxstaens, G., Kahrilas, P. J., & Logemann J. A. (2009). Relationship between manometric and videofluoroscopic measures of swallow function in healthy adults and patients treated for head and neck cancer with various modalities. *Dysphagia, 24*(2), 196–203.

Pauloski, B. R., Rademaker, A. W., Logemann, J. A., Stein, D., Beery, Q., Newman, L., . . . MacCracken, E. (2000). Pretreatment swallowing function in patients with head and neck cancer. *Head & Neck, 22*(5), 474–482.

Pawełczyk, A., Kotlicka-Antczak, M., Łojek, E., Ruszpel, A., & Pawełczyk, T. (2018). Schizophrenia patients have higher-order language and extralinguistic impairments, *Schizophrenia Research, 192,* 274–280.

Pawełczyk, A., Pawełczyk, T., Łojek, E., Żurner, N., & Gawłowska-Sawosz, M. (2018). Higher-order language dysfunctions as a possible neurolinguistic endophenotype for schizophrenia: Evidence from patients and their unaffected first degree relatives. *Psychiatry Research, 267,* 63–72. https://doi.org/10.1016/j.psychres .2018.05.070

Paxton, A. (2013). *On lumpectomy surgical margins, a push for clarity.* Retrieved from http://www .captodayonline.com/Archives/1012/1012b_ lumpectomy_surgical.html

Peterson, K., & Fenn, J. (2005). Treatment of dysphagia and dysphonia following skull base surgery. *Otolaryngologic Clinics of North America, 38*(4), 809–817.

Pitts, L. L., Morales, S., & Stierwalt, J. A. G. (2018). Lingual pressure as a clinical indicator of swallow function in Parkinson's disease. *Journal of Speech, Language, and Hearing Research, 61,* 257–265.

Plowman, E., Watts, S., Tabor, L., Robison, R., Gaziano, J., Domer, A., . . . Gooch, C. (2016). Impact of expiratory strength training in amyotrophic lateral sclerosis. *Muscle Nerve, 54*(1), 48–53.

Ponsford, J., Facem, P., Willmott, C., Rothwell, A., Kelly, A., Nelms, R., & Ng, K. (2004). Use of the Westmead PTA scale to monitor recovery of memory after mild head injury. *Brain Injury*, *18*(6), 603–614.

Pratt, C., Hopf, R., & Larriba-Quest, K. (2017). Characteristics of individuals with autism spectrum disorder (ASD). *The Reporter*, *21*(17). Retrieved from https://www.iidc.indiana.edu/pages/characteristics

Prohaska, C. C., Nordon-Craft, A., Gallagher, M., Burnham, E. L., Clark, B. J., Ho, M., . . . Moss, M. (2017). Critical care: Improving ICU exercise, rehabilitation, recovery, and survivorship: Patterns of utilization and effects of hospital-specific factors on physical, occupational, and speech therapy for critically ill patients with acute respiratory failure: Results of a five-year national sample. *American Journal of Respiratory and Critical Care Medicine*, *195*. Retrieved from https://search.proquest.com/docview/1926870593

Prosiegel, M., Schelling, A., & Wagner-Sonntag, E. (2004). Dysphagia and multiple sclerosis. *The International MS Journal*, *11*, 22–31.

Pulvermuller, F., Neininger, B., Elbert, T., Mohr, B., Rockstroh, B., Koebbel, P., & Taub, E. (2001). Constraint-induced therapy of chronic aphasia after stroke. *Stroke*, *32*, 1621–1626.

Raju, K., & Coombe-Jones, M. (2015). An overview of delirium for the community and hospital clinician. *Progress in Neurology and Psychiatry*, *19*(6), 23–27. https://doi.org/10.1002/pnp.406

Rangarathnam, B., & McCullough, G. (2017). Swallowing exercises in patients post-stroke: What is the current evidence? *Perspectives of the ASHA Special Interest Groups (SIG 13)*, *2*(1), 4–12.

Rihn, A., Kane, J., Albert, J., Vacaro, A. R., & Hilibrand, A. S. (2011). What is the incidence and severity of dysphagia after anterior cervical surgery? *Clinical Orthopaedics and Related Research*, *3*, 658–665.

Ringen, P. A., Engh, J. A., Birkenaes, A. B., Andreassen, O. A., & Andreassen, O. A. (2014). Increased mortality in schizophrenia due to cardiovascular disease—a non-systematic review of epidemiology, possible causes and interventions. *Frontiers in Psychiatry*. https://doi.org/10.3389/fpsyt.2014.00137

Rinkel, R. N., Verdonck-de Leeuw, I. M., de Bree, R., Aaronson, N. K., & Leemans, C. R. (2015).

Validity of patient-reported swallowing and speech outcomes in relation to objectively measured oral function among patients treated for oral or oropharyngeal cancer. *Dysphagia*, *30*(2), 196–204.

Rinkel, R. N., Verdonck-de Leeuw, I. M., van Reij, E. J., Aaronson, N. K., & Leemans, C. R. (2008). Speech handicap index in patients with oral and pharyngeal cancer: Better understanding of patients' complaints. *Head & Neck*, *30*(7), 868–874.

Robbins, J., Kays, S., Gangnon, R., Hind, J., Hewitt, A., Gentry, L., & Taylor, A. (2007). The effects of lingual exercise in stroke patients with dysphagia. *Archives of Physical Medicine and Rehabilitation*, *88*, 150–158.

Robbins, J., Levine, R., Maser, A., Rosenbek, J., & Kempster, G. (1993). Swallowing after unilateral stroke of the cerebral cortex. *Archives of Physical Medicine and Rehabilitation*, *74*, 1295–1300.

Rogus-Pulia, N., Malandraki, G., Johnson, S., & Robbins, J. (2015). Understanding dysphagia in dementia: The present and the future. *Current Physical Medicine Rehabilitation Reports*, *3*, 86–97.

Ross, E. D., Orbelo, D. M., Cartwright, J., Hansel, S., Burgard, M., Testa, J. A., & Buck, R. (2001). Affective-prosodic deficits in schizophrenia: Comparison to patients with brain damage and relation to schizophrenic symptoms [corrected]. *Journal of Neurology, Neurosurgery, and Psychiatry*, *70*(5), 597– 604.

Ruegg, S., Hagen, M., Hohl, U., Kappos, L., Fuhr, P., Plasilov, M., . . . Heinimann, K. (2005). Oculopharyngeal muscular dystrophy—an underdiagnosed disorder? *Swiss Medical Weekly*, *135*, 574–586.

Sagi, C., Beutler, W., Carroll, E., & Connolly, J. (2002). Airway complications associated with surgery on the anterior cervical spine. *Spine*, *27*, 949–953.

Salama, J. K., Stenson, K. M., Kistner, E. O., Mittal, B. B, Argiris, A., Witt, M. E., . . . Vokes, E. E. (2008). Induction chemotherapy and concurrent chemoradiotherapy for locoregionally advanced head and neck cancer: A multiinstitutional phase II trial investigating three radiotherapy dose levels. *Annals of Oncology*, *19*(10), 1787–1794.

Salama, J. K., Stenson, K. M., List, M. A., Mell, L. K., Maccracken, E., Cohen, E. E., . . . Haraf, D. J. (2008). Characteristics associated with swallowing changes after concurrent chemotherapy and radiotherapy in patients with head and neck cancer. *Archives of Otolaryngology-Head & Neck Surgery*, *134*(10), 1060–1065.

Salat, D., Robinson, M., Miller, D., Clark, D., & McGlinchey, R. (2017). Neuroimaging of deployment-associated traumatic brain injury (TBI) with a focus on mild TBI (mTBI) since 2009. *Brain Injury*, *31*(9), 1204–1219.

Salghetti A., & Martinuzzi A (2012). Dysphagia in cerebral palsy. *Eastern Journal of Medicine*, *17*, 188–193.

Sapir, S., Spielman, J., Ramig, L., Story, B., & Fox, C. (2007). Effects of intensive voice treatment (the Lee Silverman Voice Treatment [LSVT]) on vowel articulation in dysarthric individuals with idiopathic Parkinson disease: Acoustic and perceptual findings. *Journal of Speech, Language, and Hearing Research*, *50*, 899–912.

Saravanan G., Ranganathan V., Gandhi A., & Jaya V. (2016). Speech outcome in oral cancer patients—pre- and post-operative evaluation: A cross-sectional study. *Indian Journal of Palliative Care*, *22*(4), 499–503.

Schölderlen T., Staiger, A., Lampe, R., & Ziegler, W. (2013). Dysarthria syndromes in adult cerebral palsy. *Journal of Medical Speech*, *20*(4), 100–105.

Schreck, K. A., Williams, K., & Smith, A. F. (2004). A comparison of eating behaviors between children with and without autism. *Journal of Autism and Developmental Disorders*, *34*, 433–438.

Schreiber, J. E., Possin, K. L., Girard, J. M., & Rey-Casserly, C. (2014). Executive function in children with attention deficit/hyperactivity disorder: The NIH EXAMINER battery. *Journal of the International Neuropsychological Society*, *20*(1), 41–51. https://doi.org/10.1017/S13556 17713001100

Sharma, P., Eesa, M., & Scott, J. (2009). Toxic and metabolic encephalopathies. *American Journal of Roentenology*, *193*, 879–886.

Sharpe, G., Camoes Costa, V., Doubé, W., Sita, J., McCarthy, C., & Carding, P. (2018). Communication changes with laryngectomy and impact on quality of life: A review. *Quality of Life Research*. Advance online publication. Retrieved from https://doi.org/10.1007/s11136-018-2033-y

Shores, E., Marosszeky, J., Sandanam, J., & Batchelor, J. (1986). Preliminary validation of a scale for measuring the duration of post-traumatic amnesia. *Medical Journal of Australia*, *144*, 569–572.

Sima, A., Zhang, W., Muzik, O., Kreipke, C., Rafols, J., & Hoffman, W. (2009). Sequential abnormalities in Type 1 diabetic encephalopathy and the effects of C-peptide. *Review of Diabetic Studies*, *6*(3), 211–222.

Simpson, S., Blizzard, L., Otahal, P., Van der Mei, I., & Taylor, B. (2011). Latitude is significantly associated with the prevalence of multiple sclerosis: A meta-analysis. *Journal of Neurology, Neurosurgery, and Psychiatry*, *82*, 1132–1141. https://doi.org/10.1136/jnnp.2011.240432

Smith, D. J., Langan, J., McLean, G., Guthrie, B., & Mercer, S. W. (2013). Schizophrenia is associated with excess multiple physical-health comorbidities but low levels of recorded cardiovascular disease in primary care: Cross-sectional study. *BMJ Open*, *3*(4). https://doi .org/10.1136/bmjopen-2013–002808

Smith-Hammond, A., New, C., Pietrobon, R., Curtis, D. J., Scharver, C. H., & Turner, D. A. (2004). Prospective analysis of incidence and risk factors of dysphagia in spine surgery patients: Comparison of anterior cervical, posterior cervical, and lumbar procedures. *Spine*, *13*, 1441–1446.

Smits, L. L., van Harten, A. C., Pijnenburg, Y. A. L., Koedam, E., Bouwman, F. H., Sistermans, N., . . . van der Flier, W. M. (2015). Trajectories of cognitive decline in different types of dementia. *Psychological Medicine*, *45*(5), 1051–1059.

Sparks, R., Helm, N., & Albert, M. (1974). Aphasia rehabilitation resulting from melodic intonation therapy. *Cortex*, *10*, 303–316.

Spencer, K. A., & Brown, K. (2018). Dysarthria following stroke. *Seminars in Speech and Language*, *39*, 15–24.

Sprich, S. E., Safren, S. A., Finkelstein, D., Remmert, J. E., & Hammerness, P. (2016). A randomized controlled trial of cognitive behavioral therapy for ADHD in medication treated adolescents. *Journal of Child Psychology and Psychiatry, 57*(11), 1218–1226.

Starmer, H., Gourin, C. Lua, L. L., & Burkhead, L. (2011). Pretreatment swallowing assessment in head and neck cancer patients, *Laryngoscope, 121*(6), 1208–1211.

Starmer, M., Tippett, D., Webster, K., Quon, H., Jones, B., Hardy, S., & Gourin, G. (2014). Swallowing outcomes in patients with oropharyngeal cancer undergoing organ-preservation treatment. *Head & Neck, 36*(10), 1392–1397. https://doi.org/10.1002/hed.23465

Steidl, E., Ribeiro, C., Gonçalves, B., Fernandes, N., Antunes, V., & Mancopes, R. (2015). Relationship between dysphagia and exacerbations in chronic obstructive pulmonary disease: A literature review. *International Archives of Otorhinolaryngology, 19*(1), 74. https://doi.org/10.1055/s-0034-1376430

Stone, M., Langguth, M., Woo, J., Chen, H., & Prince, L. (2014). Tongue motion patterns in post-glossectomy and typical speakers: A principal components analysis. *Journal of Speech, Language, and Hearing Research, 57*(3), 707–717.

St. George, R. J., Nutt, J. G., Burchiel, K. J., & Horak, F. B. (2010). A meta-regression of the long-term effects of deep brain stimulation on balance and gait in PD. *Neurology, 75*(14), 1292–1299.

Suarez-Cunqueiro, M., Schramm, A., Schoen, R., Seoane-Lestón, J., Otero-Cepeda, X. L., Bormann, K. H., . . . Gellrich, N. C. (2008). Speech and swallowing impairment after treatment for oral and oropharyngeal cancer. *Archives of Otolaryngology-Head & Neck Surgery, 134*(12), 1299–1304.

Sun, J-H., Tan, L., & Yu, J-T. (2014). Post-stroke cognitive impairment: Epidemiology, mechanisms and management. *Annals of Translation Medicine, 2*(8), 80.

Suntrup, S., Kemmling, A., Warnecke, T., Hamacher, C., Oelenberg, T., Niederstadt, T., . . . Dziewas, R. (2015). The impact of lesion location on dysphagia incidence, pattern, and complications in acute stroke. Part 1: Dysphagia incidence, severity, and aspiration. *European Journal of Neurology, 22*, 832–838.

Swan, K., Hopper, M., Wenke, R., Jackson, C., Till, T., & Conway, E. (2018). Speech-language pathologist interventions for communication in moderate–severe dementia: A systematic review. *American Journal of Speech Language Pathology, 27*, 836–852.

Tariq, S., Tumosa, N., Chibnall, J., Perry, H., & Morley, J. (2006). The Saint Louis University Mental Status (SLUMS) Examination for detecting mild cognitive impairment and dementia is more sensitive than the Mini-Mental Status Examination (MMSE)—a pilot study. *American Journal of Geriatric Psychiatry, 14*, 900–910.

Tasli, H., Eser, B., Basik, B., & Birkent, H. (2018). Does pepsin play a role in etiology of laryngeal nodules? *Journal of Voice*. Advance online publication. https://doi.org/10.1016/j.jvoice.2018.04.009

Tassorelli, C., Bergamaschi, R., Buscone, S., Bartolo, M., Furnari, A., Crivelli, P . . . Nappi, G. (2008). Dysphagia in multiple sclerosis: From pathogenesis to diagnosis. *Neurological Sciences, 29*, S360–S363.

Tauber, S., Staszewski, O., Prinz, M., Weis, J., Nolte, K., Bunkowski, S., . . . Nau, R. (2016). HIV encephalopathy: Glial activation and hippocampal neuronal apoptosis, but limited neural repair. *HIV Medicine, 17*, 143–151.

Teasdale, G., & Jennett, B. (1974). Assessment of coma and impaired consciousness: A practical scale. *Lancet, 2*(7872), 81–84.

Teismann, I., Warnecke, T., Suntrup, S., Steinstrater, O., Kronenberg, L., Ringelstein, E., . . . Dziewas, R. (2011). Cortical Processing of Swallowing in ALS patients with progressive dysphagia—A magnetoencephalographic study. *PLoS One, 6*(5), e19987.

Thakur, K., Motta, M., Asemota, A., Kirsch, H., Benavides, D., Schneider, E., . . . Venkatesan, A. (2013). Predictors of outcome in acute encephalitis. *Neurology, 81*(9), 793–800.

Theander, K., Hasselgren, M., Luhr, K., Eckerblad, J., Unosson, M., & Karlsson, I. (2014). Symptoms and impact of symptoms on function and health in patients with chronic obstructive pulmonary disease and chronic heart failure in primary health care. *International Journal of*

Chronic Obstructive Pulmonary Disease, 9, 785–794. https://doi.org/10.2147/COPD.S62563

The Challenge of Neurodegenerative Diseases. (n.d.). Retrieved from https://neurodiscovery.harvard.edu/challenge

Trenova, A., Slavov, G., Manova, M., Aksentieva, J., Miteva, L., & Stanilova, S. (2016). Cognitive impairment in multiple sclerosis. *Folia Medica, 58*(3), 157–163.

Troche, M., Okun, M. S., Rosenbek, J. C., Musson, N., Fernandez, H. H., Rodriquez, R., . . . Sapienza, C. M. (2010). Aspiration and swallowing in Parkinson disease and rehabilitation with EMST: A randomized trial. *Neurology, 75,* 1912–1919.

Turner, M. R., Al-Chalabi, A., Chio, A., Hardiman, O., Kiernan, M. C., Rohrer, J. D., . . . Talbot, K. (2017). Genetic screening in sporadic ALS and FTD. *Journal of Neurology, Neurosurgery, and Psychiatry, 88,* 1042–1044. https://doi.org/10.1136/jnnp-2017-315995

Tyler, K. (2004). Update on herpes simplex encephalitis. *Reviews in Neurological Diseases, 1*(4), 169–178.

Vaezi M. F., Hicks D. M., Abelson T., & Richter, J. E. (2003). Laryngeal signs and symptoms and gastroesophageal reflux disease (GERD): A critical assessment of cause and effect association. *Clinical Gastroenterology and Hepatology, 1*(5), 333–344.

Valk, J., & van der Knaap, S. (1992). Toxic encephalopathy. *American Journal of Neuroradiolgy, 13,* 747–760.

van Eijck, M. M., Schoonman, G. G., van der Naalt, J., de Vries, J., & Roks, G. (2018). Diffuse axonal injury after traumatic brain injury is a prognostic factor for functional outcome: A systematic review and meta-analysis. *Brain Injury, 32*(4), 395–402. https://doi.org/10.1080/02699052.2018.1429018

van den Engel-Hoek, L., Erasmus, C., Hendriks, J., Geurts, A., Klein, W., Pillen, S., . . . de Groot, I. (2013). Oral muscles are progressively affected in Duchenne muscular dystrophy: Implications for dysphagia treatment. *Journal of Neurology, 260,* 1295–1303.

van der Molen, M. A. Rossum, A. H. Ackerstaff, A. H., Smeele, L.E., Rasch, C. R., & Hilgers, F. J. (2009). Pretreatment organ function in patients with advanced head and neck cancer: Clinical outcome measures and patients' views, *BMC Ear Nose Throat Disorders, 9,* 10.

Venkatesan, A. (2015). Epidemiology and outcomes of acute encephalitis. *Current Opinion in Neurology, 28*(3), 277–282.

Venkatesan, A., Tunkel, A., Bloch, K., Lauring, A., Sejvar, J., & Bitnun, A. (2013). Case definitions, diagnostic algorithms, and priorities in encephalitis: Consensus statement of the International Encephalitis Consortium. *Clinical Infectious Diseases, 57*(8), 1114–1128.

Venkateswaran, S., & Shevell, M. (2008). Comorbidities and clinical determinants of outcome in children with spastic quadriplegic cerebral palsy. *Developmental Medicine & Child Neurology, 50,* 216–222.

Walker, W., Ketchum, J., Marwitz, J., Chen, T., Hammond, F., Sherer, M., & Meythaler, J. (2010). A multicentre study on the clinical utility of post-traumatic amnesia duration in predicting global outcome after moderate-severe traumatic brain injury. *Journal of Neurology, Neurosurgery, and Psychiatry, 81,* 87–89.

Walshe, M. (2014). Oropharyngeal dysphagia in neurodegenerative disease. *Journal of Gastroenterology and Hepatology Research, 3*(10), 1265–1271.

Wambaugh, J., Nessler, C., Wright, S., & Mauszycki, S. (2014). Sound production treatment: Effects of blocked and random practice. *American Journal of Speech-Language Pathology, 23,* S225–S245.

Watson, B., Aizawa, L., Savundranayagam, M., & Orange, J. (2013). Links among communication, dementia and caregiver burden. *Canadian Journal of Speech-Language Pathology and Audiology, 36*(4), 276–283.

Weissenborn, K., Ennen, J., Schomerus, H., Rueckert, N., & Hecker, H. (2001). Neuropsychological characterization of hepatic encephalopathy. *Journal of Hepatology, 34,* 768–773.

Welch, K. A., & Carson, A. J. (2018). When psychiatric symptoms reflect medical conditions. *Clinical Medicine, 18*(1), 80–87. https://doi.org/10.7861/clinmedicine.18-1-80

Wilcox, M., Brummel, N., Archer, K., Ely, E., Jackson, J., & Hopkins, R. (2013). Cognitive dysfunction in ICU patients: Risk factors, predictors, and rehabilitation interventions. *Criti-*

cal Care Medicine, 41(9 Suppl. 1), S98. https://doi.org/10.1097/CCM.0b013e3182a16946

Woodson, G. E. (1993). Configuration of the glottis in laryngeal paralysis. I: Clinical study. *Laryngoscope, 103*(11, Pt 1), 1227–1234.

World Health Organization. (2014). *International classification of functioning, disability and health.* Geneva, Switzerland: Author. Retrieved from http://www.who.int/classifications/icf/en/

Xu, J., He, S., Han, Y., Pan, J., & Cao, L. (2017). Effects of modified pulmonary rehabilitation on patients with moderate to severe chronic obstructive pulmonary disease: A randomized controlled trial. *International Journal of Nursing Sciences, 4*(3), 219–224.

Ylvisaker, M., Turkstra, L., & Coelho, C. (2005). Behavioral and social interventions for individuals with traumatic brain injury: A summary of the research with clinical implications. *Seminars in Speech and Language, 26,* 256–267.

Yoder, P., Camarata, S., & Woynaroski, T. (2016). Treating comprehensibility in students with Down syndrome. *Journal of Speech, Language, and Hearing Research, 59,* 446–459.

Yorkston, K. M., Beukelman, D. R., Strand, E. A., & Hakel, M. (2010). *Management of motor speech disorders in children and adults* (3rd ed.). Austin, TX: Pro-Ed.

Yourganov, G., Smith, K., Fridriksson, J., & Rorden, C. (2015). Predicting aphasia type from brain damage measured with structural MRI. *Cortex, 73,* 203–215.

Zauner, C., Gendo, A., Kramer, L., Kranz, A., Grimm, G., & Madl, C. (2000). Metabolic encephalopathy in critically ill patients suffering from septic or nonseptic multiple organ failure. *Critical Care Medicine, 28*(5), 1310–1315.

Zerninski, R., Zini, A., & Sgan-Cohen, H. D. (2010). Lip cancer: Incidence, trends, histology and survival: 1970–2006. *British Journal of Dermatology, 162,* 1103–1109.

Ziaja, M. (A2013). Septic encephalopathy. *Current Neurological and Neuroscience Reports, 13,* 383.

Zuccalà, G., Onder, G., Pedone, C., Cocchi, A., Carosella, L., Cattel, C., . . . Bernabei, R. (2001). Cognitive dysfunction as a major determinant of disability in patients with heart failure: results from a multicentre survey. *Journal of Neurology, Neurosurgery, and Psychiatry. 70*(1), 109–112.

Zuccalà, G., Pedone, C., Cesari, M., Onder, G., Pahor, M., Marzetti, E., . . . Bernabei, R. (2003). The effects of cognitive impairment on mortality among hospitalized patients with heart failure. *American Journal of Medicine, 115*(2), 97–103.

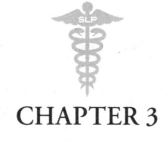

CHAPTER 3

A Guide to Neuroimaging for the Medical Speech-Language Pathologist

Linda I. Shuster

INTRODUCTION

The technologies for studying the brain in living humans have progressed at a remarkable pace, particularly in the late 20th and early 21st centuries. This progress was further advanced by U.S. government-funded or cofunded initiatives, such as the Human Connectome Project and the 2013 BRAIN Initiative. The Human Connectome Project was designed to map all of the neural connections in the human brain, whereas the mission of the BRAIN Initiative is to develop a better understanding of the typical brain, as well as to improve prevention and treatment of brain disorders, including the development of cures. Although the research efforts in this arena have been notable (a search of PubMed using the phrase "magnetic resonance imaging" resulted in 27,303 results in 2017 alone), the potential for the clinical translation of these efforts has received insufficient attention in the research literature (Shuster, 2018; Ward, 2015a, 2015b). As a result, clinical brain imaging, although still impressive, has

lagged behind research imaging. For example, many researchers have sought to identify brain biomarkers for predicting recovery from aphasia after a stroke; however, the clinical utility and applicability of these biomarkers is almost never addressed in research studies (Shuster, 2018). There are, however, a variety of imaging techniques that are used clinically for the diagnosis of neurologic disorders that affect communication, and those techniques are the topic of this chapter.

Speech-language pathologists (SLPs) should understand neuroimaging techniques for a variety of reasons. One is that knowledge of changes in the brain observed through neuroimaging can help the SLP understand changes in a patient's communication and swallowing abilities over time. For example, rapidly deteriorating abilities and/or the appearance of new problems may be due to the progression of a fast-growing tumor, which can be observed through imaging. Neuroimaging results can also help the SLP to comprehend the pattern of behavioral deficits the patient is demonstrating and can serve as an additional resource for shaping prognostic decisions. In addition, SLPs are often in the position of having to help patients and their families understand the neuroimaging results. Finally, many researchers have suggested that neuroimaging data could be used to support decisions regarding candidacy for speech and language therapy or for a particular therapy approach. It is likely that the task of explaining imaging-related treatment decisions would fall to the SLP, so it is critical that he or she understand the techniques, their strengths, and their weaknesses (Shuster, 2018).

Neuroimaging Quality

There are several important parameters related to the quality of information that can be obtained from neuroimaging: temporal resolution, spatial resolution, signal-to-noise ratio (SNR), contrast, and the presence or absence of artifacts. Resolution refers to the detail that can be observed through imaging techniques, either with regard to time, as in temporal resolution, or with regard to location, as in spatial resolution.

Neural events in the brain occur on a time scale of milliseconds (e.g., Diba, Amarasingham, Mizuseki, & Buzsáki, 2014). Temporal resolution of an imaging method refers to the time scale at which it can capture changes in brain function (Zani, Biella, & Proverbio, 2012). Neuroimaging methods that can image brain function at time scales that are closer to the time scale of real-time brain events (such as the generation of neuronal action potentials and post-synaptic potentials) are said to have better temporal resolution than those that obtain information on a scale that is longer than real-time brain events.

Although not often acknowledged, spatial resolution can have two meanings (Papanicolaou, 2017). The most commonly used meaning refers to the minimum size of a brain region (typically, in millimeters) that can be differentiated from another brain region. This type of spatial resolution is measured in a unit called the pixel (picture element) for two-dimensional images or the voxel (volume element) for a three-dimensional image. The second meaning of spatial resolution, which applies specifically to studies of brain function rather than studies of structure, refers to the maximum number of brain regions whose level of activity can be observed at a given time.

Signal-to-noise ratio is a measure of the level of the signal of interest relative to the level of background noise (Welvaert & Rosseel, 2013). Because this is a ratio, the higher the level of noise, the more difficult it will be to detect the signal, especially if the signal is small. There are a variety of noise sources in neuroimaging, including the machines that are used to generate the images, as well as the physiological noise that comes from the patient him- or herself. Images with higher SNR will be of better quality than those with lower SNR.

Image contrast (or contrast-to-noise ratio, CNR) is similar to SNR. However, whereas SNR reflects a measure of the raw signal in the context of background noise, contrast refers to differences in signal intensity between different tissues. For example, when the contrast is good, brain gray matter and brain white matter can be clearly differentiated. Contrast can be created by agents that are already present in the body (i.e., an endogenous agent) or by the intravenous injection of a contrast agent into the body, (i.e., an exogenous agent).

Finally, image quality may be affected by artifacts. Artifacts arise from a variety of sources, but they all diminish the quality of the image. One source of artifact is movement of different types. When people move their heads in a magnetic resonance imaging scanner, this can decrease the quality of the image. If the movement is small, it is possible to apply corrections to improve the image quality; however, if the head movement is large, the images must be discarded. Similarly, patients cannot speak during the collection of electro-encephalographic (EEG) data, because the muscle movement involved in speaking will generate electrical artifacts that decrease the quality of the EEG recording.

In summary, the quality of neuroimaging data is affected by a variety of factors, and the nature of the effect of these factors on image quality differs for different neuroimaging modalities. No neuroimaging modality is perfect, and there is always some trade-off with regard to the different aspects of quality. For example, the modality with the best temporal resolution will not provide the best spatial resolution, and vice versa. There are aspects of the imaging that can be manipulated to improve quality, but these also involve trade-offs, such as longer times for acquiring the images. In this chapter, each clinical neuroimaging modality is described, including the factors that influence image quality.

Clinical Versus Research Scanning

As noted above, there are thousands of research articles published each year that explore the use of neuroimaging to differentially diagnose, track changes in, predict recovery from, and determine risk for a variety of neurologic diseases. However, the translation of that research to clinical practice has been slow for a variety of reasons. One reason is that clinical translation is often not considered when research studies are designed; thus, there may be aspects of the study that make translation impractical or unaffordable, especially for a medical center with limited financial resources (e.g., Shuster, 2018; Ward, 2015a, 2015b). Another reason is that the process of taking a procedure from research to a billable clinical procedure is long and complex (Yousem, 2014). Thus, research studies that clinicians encounter may still be

a long way from being used in the clinical settings in which they practice. The neuroimaging modalities that are discussed in this chapter are those that are currently being used in clinical practice.

COMPUTED TOMOGRAPHY

Overview of Computed Tomography

Computed tomography (CT), also called computerized axial tomography (CAT), is one of the oldest clinical neuroimaging technologies (Bigler, 2017), and most major hospitals are equipped with CT scanners (Cierniak, 2011a, 2011b). CT uses x-rays (ionizing radiation). X-rays are effective for imaging because when they are directed into the body, different tissues attenuate the x-rays differently. In other words, the x-rays pass more easily through some tissues than others and this is the source of the contrast (Caldemeyer & Buckwalter, 1999). The greater the attenuation, the brighter the tissue appears on the x-ray image. For example, bone has higher attenuation than most tissues, which is why it appears so white in an x-ray. In CT, the patient is moved into a donut-shaped tube, or gantry, by a motorized table (Brenner & Hall, 2007). A source of x-rays is located inside the gantry and rotates around the organ of interest, for example, the brain, allowing the passage of the x-rays through the tissue at different angles. There is also a detector that rotates around the patient that detects the amount of attenuation that occurs at different locations. The images are collected as "slices" then reconstructed by a computer into 3-D images, hence the "computed" in computed tomography.

In addition to the endogenous contrast that is an inherent property of a tissue, exogenous contrast agents can be used to enhance contrast. These agents work by affecting the attenuation of the x-ray beam. For example, CT can be used to visualize arteries using CT angiography (CTA) and to image blood volume and flow through CT perfusion (CTP) (Ezzeddine et al., 2001). These studies both require the use of a contrast agent. Another factor related to image contrast is the human eye (Kim & Mukherjee, 2013). Historically, neuroimages have been read by neuroradiologists, and humans can only differentiate 60 to 80 levels of gray. Therefore, when viewing grayscale images such as those generated by structural CT, the neuroradiologist must adjust the viewing window to achieve the optimal contrast.

CT Details

As noted above, 3D images are divided into voxels, and this determines the spatial resolution of the image. The size of the voxels is controlled by factors inherent to the technology and by parameters that can be set on the scanner. One parameter is slice thickness, which determines the size of the voxel in one of the three dimensions. The parameters that determine the size of the voxels in the other two dimensions are the matrix and the field of view. The field of view refers to the size of the "window" through which the object of interest is imaged, and the matrix indicates how finely the window is divided up into smaller pieces so that the image can be viewed in greater detail. The spatial resolution of brain structural CT is on the order of 5 millimeters for slice thickness (Kim & Mukherjee, 2013), and less than a millimeter in the other two dimensions.

Artifacts in CT can be caused by several factors, including beam hardening, head motion, and a phenomenon called the partial volume effect. Beam hardening results from the fact that the x-ray is altered as it passes through the tissue (Barrett & Keat, 2004). Head motion results in blurring of the image.

Partial volume effects are due to the fact that a voxel can contain different tissue types. In order to understand this, imagine you are looking at a tree through a window, which is your field of view. This window is divided into panes, and the panes are the matrix. If you look through a given pane, you may see part of a tree branch, the sky, a house, and so forth. The data that are collected are an average of the signal coming from the voxel; thus, rather than getting pure tree signal, which is your signal of interest, you get an average of tree, sky, and house. Head motion exacerbates the partial volume effect. Think of the tree and its branches moving in the wind in and out of the pane; you see different amounts and parts of the tree through the pane at different times.

Advantages and Disadvantages of CT

There are several advantages to CT scanning. One is that the technology is less expensive than some of the other technologies, which is why smaller medical facilities can afford CT scanners. Another advantage is that there is nothing about the patient that would prevent him or her from entering the scanner environment, unlike other technologies that will be discussed later. If a patient comes into the emergency room unaccompanied, for example, they can undergo a CT scan without having to be screened for safety issues, unlike MRI. CT scans without contrast can be obtained very quickly, which is another advantage (Kamalian, Lev, & Gupta, 2016). According to the American College of Obstetrics and Gynecology, with a few exceptions, radiation exposure during clinical CT is at a dose much lower than the exposure associated with fetal harm (American College of Obstetricians and Gynecologists, 2017). Therefore, it can be used during pregnancy, although MRI is preferred when possible. Moreover, the use of contrast is not contraindicated during lactation. With that said, the ionizing radiation used in CT is a known carcinogen (Brenner & Hall, 2007; Lin, 2010). Although the risk for developing cancer from clinical CT scanning is still not completely agreed upon, it is agreed that its use should be judicious, and the justification for its use should be very clear, especially for children (Food and Drug Administration, 2018; Lin, 2010). Because it exposes the body to ionizing radiation, CT is considered to be one of the more invasive neuroimaging techniques. Another risk factor is a reaction to a contrast agent. For example, agents containing iodine provide the best contrast in CTA; however, some patients have negative reactions to the contrast agents that can occur immediately after the injection, or up to 7 days after injection. These reactions can include anaphylaxis, flushing, and cardiac manifestations (Bottinor, Polkampally, & Jovin, 2013).

Clinical Uses of CT

CT is used for a variety of clinical purposes. Noncontrast CT is typically the first neuroimaging procedure conducted when a patient comes into the emergency room with a suspected stroke (Birenbaum, Bancroft, & Felsberg, 2011; Mair & Wardlaw, 2014). This is often followed by CTP to determine how well the brain is perfused, (i.e., whether there is an adequate blood supply), and/or CTA for imaging the vasculature (Dorn et al., 2012; Munich, Shakir, & Snyder 2016). CT with contrast also is very useful for detecting tumors, for example, in the larynx (Liguori et al., 2015), and the brain (Fink, Muzi, Peck, & Krohn, 2015). These different imaging techniques are referred to as modalities, and when several of these (CT, CTP, CTA) are employed with a patient, it is referred to as multimodal imaging (Powers et al., 2018). Figure 3–1 shows a CT image in the axial plane of a woman with an intracerebral and intraventricular hemorrhage.

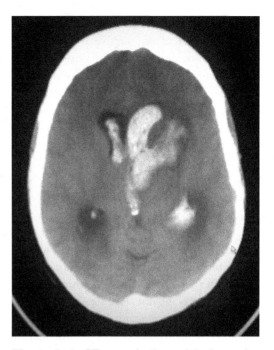

Figure 3–1. CT scan in the axial plane of a young woman with an intracerebral and intraventricular hemorrhage, one week postpartum. The bright white areas within the brain indicate the presence of acute blood. *Source:* https://en.wikipedia.org/wiki/Intracerebral_hemorrhage. This work has been released into the public domain by its author, Glitzy queen00 at the Wikipedia project. This applies worldwide. Glitzy queen00 grants anyone the right to use this work for any purpose, without any conditions, unless such conditions are required by law.

POSITRON EMISSION TOMOGRAPHY

Overview of Positron Emission Tomography

Whereas CT is essentially a view of brain structure, positron emission tomography (PET) provides information about brain function. In particular, it provides images of brain functions, such as blood volume and flow, and the binding of neurotransmitters to their receptors (Muehllenher & Karp, 2006; Politis

& Piccini, 2012; Workman & Coleman, 2006). In PET, a radioactive tracer (radiotracer) is introduced into the patient, typically through injection into the bloodstream. Imaging methods that employ radiotracers, such as PET, are types of nuclear medicine. It is called nuclear medicine because important events that lead to the ability to produce the images take place in the atomic nucleus of the radiotracer (Baghaei, Wong, & Li, 2013). The radiotracers used most often in PET contain radioisotopes of the elements carbon, nitrogen, and oxygen, or fluorine. The radiotracers typically are made in a machine called a cyclotron, which is expensive and requires expertise in working with radioactivity, which is why PET scanners are not as ubiquitous as CT scanners (Politis & Piccini, 2012). The radiotracers are used to "tag" or "label" biologically important molecules, such as water, glucose, or neurotransmitters.

PET produces functional maps, and in order to provide better localization of function, the PET maps are overlaid on structural images, something that is referred to as coregistration. Up until 2000, this was accomplished most often by acquiring a separate CT scan. However, this posed challenges for trying to accurately align the two scans, and in 2000, combined PET/CT machines became available that are mostly what is sold today (Baghaei et al., 2013). PET images are also sometimes coregistered with MRI images (Politis & Piccini, 2012).

PET Details

Radioactive elements are unstable and, as a result, undergo decay, which is a loss of energy from the nucleus. In the tracers used for PET, this involves the decay of the protons into neutrons, neutrinos, and positrons. The positron travels a short distance out of the nucleus, (hence the phrase, *positron emission*) and even-

tually encounters an electron, at which point both are annihilated. This annihilation event releases a pair of photons traveling in opposite directions. It is critical that two photons that are generated be detected within a short time of one another (a phenomenon termed coincidence) in order for the event to be localized within the brain, and the PET hardware, which involves detectors/cameras that encircle the brain, is constructed so as to be able to detect these coinciding events. Thus, PET is an indirect measure of function, because it is mapping the location of the radiotracer rather than directly imaging brain function, such as when electrodes are placed directly into nerve cells (Lameka, Farwell, & Ichise, 2016). Radiotracer decay rate is described by its half-life, which is the time it takes for half of the substance to decay (Turkington, 2011), and different radiotracers have different half-lives, some as short as a few minutes. The advantage of radiotracers with short half-lives is that patients are exposed to less radioactivity, but the disadvantage is that there must be a cyclotron on site, or the radiotracers with short half-lives would decay before they could be injected into the patient. One frequently used radiotracer, fludeoxyglucose (FDG), has a half-life of 110 minutes, so it is possible for it to be made off-site, but others are much shorter than that. Once the radiotracer is introduced into the patient, there is a waiting period while it accumulates in the tissue of interest, which can take up to an hour. Figure 3–2 shows an axial image of FDG-PET.

The spatial resolution of PET is approximately 4 to 6 mm, lower than magnetic resonance imaging (MRI) or CT (Bettinardi, Castiglioni, De Bernardi, & Gilardi, 2014; Griffeth, 2005; Lameka, Farwell, & Ichise, 2016). The spatial resolution is partly a function of the particular radiotracer and how far the positron travels before it is annihilated. Thus, in addition to its half-life, another important feature of a radiotracer is that it has

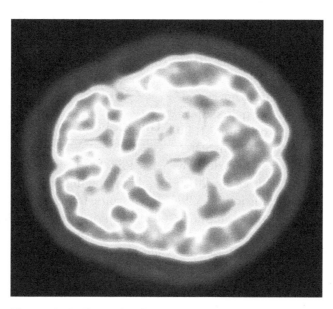

Figure 3–2. Example of a positron emission tomography (PET) axial scan of a 56-year-old male. Darker areas show more accumulated tracer substance (FDG) and lighter areas are regions where low to no tracer has accumulated. Normally, the image would be encoded in color. *Source:* https://commons.wikimedia.org/wiki/File:PET-image.jpg. This work has been released into the public domain by its author, Jens Maus. This applies worldwide. Jens Maus grants anyone the right to use this work for any purpose, without any conditions, unless such conditions are required by law.

low energy decay (the amount of energy determines how far the positron travels). The temporal resolution of PET is tens of seconds up to minutes (Zani, Biella, & Proverbio, 2003; updated in 2012 at https://erplabcnr.word press.com/the-lab/publications/books-book-chapters/book-chapters/). Contrast agents may be used in combined PET/CT evaluations during the CT portion to enhance anatomic localization (Antoch, Veit, Bockisch, & Kuehl, 2011 Cronin, Prakesh, & Blake, 2010).

There are a variety of sources of artifact in PET that must be addressed. These include partial volume effects, head motion, and attenuation, or the loss of coincidence events (Bettinardi et al., 2014; Kawaguchi, Tateishi, Inuoe, & Kim, 2013; Soret, Bacharach, & Buvat, 2007; Turkington, 2011). These artifacts can

be corrected to some extent. For example, an advantage of combined PET/CT is that the CT scan provides a more effective means for addressing attenuation than methods used in stand-alone PET scanners, although there are some drawbacks to this approach (Kawaguchi, Tateishi, Inoue, & Kim, 2013; Mawlawi, Wendt, & Wong, 2013). However, the use of a contrast agent during the CT scan can negatively affect attenuation correction (Antoch et al., 2011).

Advantages and Disadvantages of PET

One advantage of PET is that it provides information about brain function. In particular, it can provide information about brain metabolism, changes in regional blood volume and flow, and the binding of neurotransmitters to their receptors (Politis & Piccini, 2012). There are several disadvantages to PET. As mentioned earlier, PET imaging is not as readily available as CT because it re-quires expensive facilities. There are approximately 1600 PET/CT scanners in the United States, whereas in 2016 there were approximately 13,500 CT scanners (Ehman et al., 2017; https://www.statista.com/statistics/266539/distribution-of-equipment-for-computer-tomography/). Another disadvantage is that it involves exposing the patient to radioactivity. The amount is less than in CT, but now that

PET/CT scanners are the standard, the radiation dose from the PET must be added to that of the CT when calculating radiation exposure (Lameka, Farwell, & Ichise, 2016).

Clinical Uses of PET

PET has become the standard clinical tool for staging, restaging, and monitoring response to treatment for a variety of different tumor types, including brain tumors. Figure 3–3 shows an axial PET image of glucose metabolism and the presence of a malignant brain tumor. This is one of the few

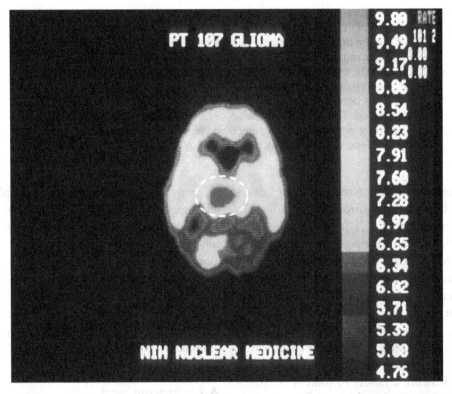

Figure 3–3. PET image in the axial plane showing glucose metabolism. The circled spot reveals a malignant brain tumor. It would appear red on actual PET scans (which are viewed as color images) because the tumor has a high rate of glucose metabolism. *Source:* https://visualsonline.cancer.gov/details.cfm?imageid=2322. Dr. Giovanni Di Chiro, Neuroimaging Section, National Institute of Neurological Disorders and Stroke, National Institutes of Health, United States Department of Health and Human Services.

uses covered by third party payers (Zhu, Lee, & Shim, 2011). Another use that is frequently covered is for presurgical planning in epilepsy (Cendes, Theodore, Brinkmann, Sulc, & Cascino, 2016). In focal epilepsy, PET is used to identify the locus of the seizures. It is also used to help identify cortex involved in language and cognition, so that the surgeon can attempt to avoid ablating those regions during surgery for tumors or epilepsy (Gerard, Tan, McKhann, & Byrne, 2016). A PET radiotracer was developed for the purpose of detecting beta amyloid and diagnosing Alzheimer's disease; however, most insurers, including Medicare, consider this use investigational and currently do not cover it. Medicare will, however, provide some coverage in the case of clinical trials aimed at investigating its utility (https://www.cms.gov/Medicare/Coverage/Coverage-with-Evidence-Development/Amyloid-PET.html).

MAGNETIC RESONANCE IMAGING

Overview of Magnetic Resonance Imaging

As the name implies, magnetism is an important component of MRI. It requires the generation of a powerful magnetic field, along with radio-frequency pulses. MRI is considered to be a noninvasive imaging technique. As in CT, the patient is moved into the MRI machine on a gantry. There are closed bore MRI machines, which look like a tube, and open bore MRI machines, which can take several configurations but have wider openings. Open bore MRI machines can reduce the feeling of claustrophobia induced by closed bore MRI, but they come at the price of a lower magnetic field strength than closed bore MRI machines. Similar to CT, there are a variety

of different imaging modalities or methods that are performed in the magnetic resonance (MR) scanner. The different modalities can image brain structure (including the arteries), brain function, white matter tracts, the brain's blood supply, and brain tissue chemical information. These modalities include structural magnetic resonance imaging, functional magnetic resonance imaging, magnetic resonance spectroscopy, diffusion-weighted imaging, and perfusion-weighted imaging. As in CT, when all or some combination of them are implemented with a given patient, this is called multimodal imaging. Multimodal MR imaging is becoming increasingly common, especially for uses such as treatment planning in acute stroke (Hao et al., 2013; Kim et al., 2014).

MRI Details

The MRI machine contains wires formed in a loop. In a new machine, an electric current is forced through the loop in a process called "ramping up." Once the magnet is ramped up, the power supply that induced the electric current can be removed without affecting the current flow, which can then be maintained for years with only minimal loss of flow. It is this current flow that generates the magnetic field used for imaging. However, to be useful for imaging, the magnetic field must be very strong. Magnetic fields are measured in a unit called tesla, abbreviated with a "T" and named after the scientist Nikola Tesla. The lowest strength MRI machines are approximately 1 T. To put this into perspective, the earth's magnetic field is approximately 0.00005 T, whereas a small bar magnet is about 0.01 T. The increased strength of the magnetic field in MRI is achieved through forming the wire into a loop, as described above. In addition, decreasing the resistance of current flow in the wire increases the strength of the magnetic field that is generated, and this decrease in resistance is achieved by using a material for the wire that has low resistance and also by cooling the wire. In modern day MRI machines, the wires are immersed in liquid helium in order to cool them. These manipulations of the wire result in what is referred to as a superconducting magnet. If you enter the MRI environment, you will see many signs that read something along the lines of "the magnetic field is always on." The only way to turn it off is to "quench" the magnet, which involves releasing the liquid helium, thus raising the temperature of the wire and decreasing the magnetic field strength. Quenching occurs only in an emergency situation, such as a fire in the room, or when the MRI machine is being decommissioned. Quenching is serious because it can produce significant damage to the coil; therefore, every imaging facility has procedures in place to determine when and how to quench the magnet.

MRI takes advantage of the fact that our bodies contain atoms that possess a characteristic called "spin" (Berger, 2002; Dale, Brown, & Semelka, 2015; Pooley, 2005). Spin can be thought of as the nucleus of the atom rotating about an axis. The rotational speed is dependent upon the particular atom, and the spins produce a small magnetic field, that is, they become small electromagnets. An important atomic nucleus for magnetic resonance imaging is the hydrogen (H) nucleus, sometimes referred to as a proton because it only contains a proton. The hydrogen proton is abundant in our bodies, both in fat and in other tissues that contain water (H_2O), such as the brain. The magnetic field generated in the MRI (B0 field) has a direction, and the direction parallel to the field is in the longitudinal or z direction (Overweg, 2006). In the common, cylindrical bore MRI machine, this direction is in the foot to head or head to foot direction. The axes of the protons' spins are typically oriented in random directions; however, when the protons (via the humans that contain them) are

placed into the B0 field, the axes of their spins either align with the B0 field or align in the opposite direction of the field (Pooley, 2005). There are slightly more protons oriented with the field than in the opposite direction, which is important. If there were equal numbers oriented in each orientation, they would cancel one another's magnetic fields out completely, but the greater number oriented with the B0 field results in what is called a net magnetization. In addition to the main magnet coil that generates the B0 field, there are other important coils in the MRI machine that produce transient perturbations of the magnetic field. Changes in the spin of the protons produced by these perturbations can be detected, and provides the basis for image formation. The MR images and image contrast are created through the manipulation of the proton net magnetization by the coils; thus, MRI can make use of endogenous contrast. The different ways of manipulating the net magnetization are referred to as pulse sequences (Parizel et al., 2010).

Although elements such as hydrogen provide an endogenous contrast, MR images are also collected using a contrast-enhancing agent. The most commonly used agents contain gadolinium, which is a paramagnetic metal (it becomes magnetized in a magnetic field; Rogosnitzky & Branch, 2016). These contrast agents highlight differences such as those between normal and pathological tissue. Like CT, MRI can be used to study the arteries via angiography (MRA), as well as to study brain perfusion. MRA can be performed with or without an exogenous contrast agent, although it is more frequently performed with a contrast agent (Hartung, Grist, & François, 2011) Brain perfusion can also be imaged using an exogenous contrast agent or taking advantage of the endogenous contrast provided by the water (H_2O) in arterial blood (arterial spin labeling, ASL). However, for a variety of reasons, MR perfusion studies have not achieved widespread clinical use outside of academic medical centers (Essig et al., 2013).

One of the important determinants of SNR in MRI is the field strength. Thus, a 3 T MRI machine has better SNR than a 1.5 T MRI machine. Other factors also affect SNR. For example, whereas it is less invasive to use ASL for MR perfusion studies as compared to injecting the patient with an exogenous contrast agent, ASL has lower SNR than contrast-enhanced perfusion imaging (Essig et al., 2013). As in CT, spatial resolution in MRI is a product of the matrix and field of view. In addition, coils are used to select "slices" of the organ of interest such as the brain. The slice thickness, along with the matrix and field of view, determines the voxel size. Higher field strength MRI machines provide better spatial resolution, because they allow for smaller voxels.

Artifacts in MRI arise from sources similar to those found in CT, and can also be due to either the hardware or the patient. Metal in the patient, such as dental braces, can produce artifacts. Like CT, MRI is sensitive to partial volume effects. Artifacts can also result from problems with the scanner, such as the B0 magnetic field not being homogeneous in the center of the scanner. It is important that the imaging facilities have a quality assurance (QA)/Quality Control program in place to ensure the system is performing optimally (Maris, 2016).

Advantages and Disadvantages of MRI

Advantages of MRI include that it has better spatial resolution than CT, and it does not involve ionizing radiation. There is no study to date that has shown a risk from noncontrast MRI, including for pregnant women (Ray, Vermeulen, Bharatha, Montanera, & Park, 2016). It can make use of the body's natural (endogenous) contrast, and it is safe

for most people to enter the scanner environment. Limitations include the potential for claustrophobia, especially in the higher field strength MRI machines that have small bores. In addition, larger patients may not fit comfortably into a smaller bore. Another limitation is that not everyone is safe to enter the magnetic field of the MRI. Patients who have certain types of metal in their bodies, such as metal slivers in their eyes from grinding metal, are not candidates for MRI. In addition, electronically activated implant devices, such as cochlear implants or cardiac pacemakers, could be damaged in the magnetic field. Some implants may be safe in a 1.5 T MRI machine, but not in a 3 T MRI machine. There are published lists that describe which devices and implants are safe and at what field strength, as well as which are not safe. In addition, some manufacturers offer guidance with regard to the MR compatibility of their devices, such as Medtronics, which produces deep brain stimulators. With regard to the use of gadolinium-based contrast agents in MR, it was initially believed that they were excreted by the body after their use. However, it has recently been shown that gadolinium can accumulate in the brain and other tissues, and the International Society for Magnetic Resonance in Medicine has provided new recommendations regarding the clinical use of gadolinium-based agents (Gulani et al., 2017; Rogosnitzky & Branch, 2016).

MRI is very sensitive to motion, so the patient must lie very still. Even then, movements such as breathing and the beating of the heart can produce artifacts (Morelli et al., 2011). Some patient motion can be tolerated, but if it is significant, the images might not be useable (Havsteen et al., 2017). In fact, it is estimated that patient movement results in an average cost to radiology departments of $115,000 per year per scanner (Andre et al., 2015). Figure 3–4 shows an MRI image affected by motion artifact.

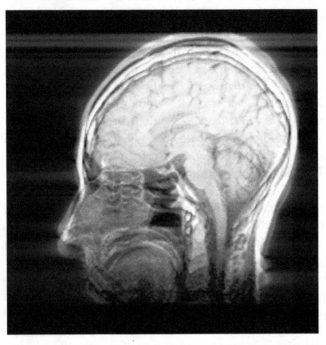

Figure 3–4. Motion artifact in an MRI sagittal image. *Source:* Image courtesy of Linda I. Shuster.

Clinical Uses of MRI

MRI is a frequently used clinical procedure. MRI with contrast is the technique of choice for imaging patients with multiple sclerosis (Alvares, Szulc, & Cheng, 2017). It is also used for detecting developmental brain abnormalities, such as Chiari II malformation, or agenesis of the corpus callosum, intracranial mass lesions, and for imaging stroke, infectious diseases, and demyelinating processes (Parizel et al., 2010). A recent development is combined PET/MRI scanning, although this has yet to see widespread clinical use. There currently are only 30 PET/MRI scanners in the United States (Ehman et al., 2017), and it is still considered investigational by most insurers. Figure 3–5 shows axial and coronal MRI images of a child who sustained an in utero stroke.

FUNCTIONAL MAGNETIC RESONANCE IMAGING

Overview of Functional Magnetic Resonance Imaging

As its name suggests, functional magnetic resonance imaging (fMRI) involves imaging brain function in the magnetic field of the MRI scanner. Generally speaking, fMRI measures brain activity by identifying changes related to blood flow while the patient performs a task. As the name also suggests, it is a measure of brain function; however, like PET, it is an *indirect* measure of function. The most common fMRI procedure images the blood oxygen level dependent (BOLD) response as a reflection of brain function. The brain needs oxygen, and there is an increased oxygen need

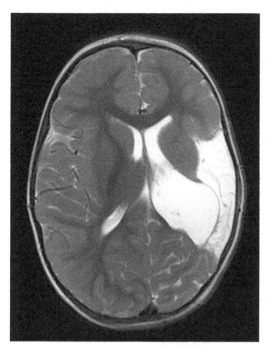 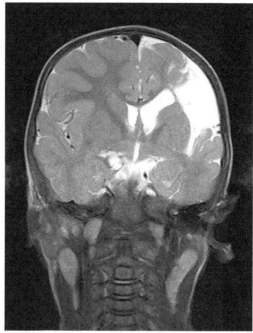

Figure 3–5. Axial and coronal MRI scans of a 17-month-old female who sustained an in utero stroke. The white area reflects encephalomalacia, which is the softening or loss of brain tissue after cerebral infarction. The term is usually used during gross pathologic inspection to describe blurred cortical margins and decreased consistency of brain tissue after infarction (Karaman, Isilkad, Yilmaz, Enver, & Albavram, 2011). Encephalomalacia is present in the distribution of the left middle cerebral artery. *Source:* Images courtesy of Kristie A. Spencer.

when neurons are active. Oxygen is delivered to neurons through the blood supply, in particular, by hemoglobin. When it is oxygenated, hemoglobin is diamagnetic, that is, it resists a magnetic field when it is placed into it. In order to deliver oxygen to neurons in the brain, the hemoglobin releases the oxygen and becomes deoxygenated. Deoxygenated hemoglobin is paramagnetic; that is, it is attracted to a magnetic field. When a region of the brain is activated, there is a brief decrease in blood oxygen as it is consumed by neurons within the region. This is followed by an increase in blood flow and the delivery of additional oxygen to the region. The BOLD signal is a function of the ratio of diamagnetic oxygenated blood to the paramagnetic deoxygenated blood (Buchbinder, 2016; Passingham & Rowe, 2016); thus, BOLD is produced by an endogenous contrast.

fMRI Details

During an fMRI scan, the patient is asked to engage in a task. A statistical analysis is used to determine the relationship between the timing of the task and the activity within brain voxels that are imaged over the course of the scan, which requires that the brain activity during the task be compared to brain activity produced during a different task or at rest. In statistics, multiple comparisons can result in the identification of false positive responses, and more comparisons result in more false positives. An fMRI scan contains information from more than 100,000 voxels, and if each voxel is compared to every other voxel, this results in massive multiple comparisons, and as many as 5000 false positives (Nichols, 2012). In fact, Bennett and colleagues put a dead Atlantic salmon into a scanner and showed it a series of photographs that depicted humans in social situations with two types of social valence, socially inclusive or socially exclusive (Bennett, Baird, Miller, & Wolford, 2010). The salmon's task was to determine what emotion the person in each photograph was experiencing. When they did not correct for multiple comparisons, they found several voxels in the dead salmon's brain that demonstrated activation in response to the task. These disappeared when they corrected for the multiple comparisons.

fMRI is subject to the same types of artifact as structural MRI, including patient head movements, partial volume effects, and patient physiological noise. It has somewhat poorer spatial resolution, on the order of 3 mm for clinical scanners, as compared to the approximately 1 mm for structural MRI (Zani et al., 2012). To improve spatial localization in fMRI, images are registered to MRI structural scans, just as PET scans are registered to CT structural scans. The temporal resolution in fMRI is relatively poor. The BOLD response lags behind the neuronal activation by as much as 6 to 8 seconds, depending on the brain region, and typical clinical scans have a temporal resolution on the order of 1 to 2 seconds (Perrin, 2013).

Advantages and Disadvantages

The advantages of fMRI are that it does not require exogenous contrast agents and, as mentioned above, there have been no problems with long-term safety identified as a result of exposure to the magnetic field of the scanner. In addition, it can be conducted during the same session in which the structural MRI is collected, which improves the quality of image registration. Disadvantages are that, as in MRI, not everyone is safe to enter the magnetic field. In addition, it requires a skilled and fairly labor-intensive computational processing stream. MRI manufacturers now sell software for presenting tasks to the patient for clinical fMRI; however, because they are prepackaged, they are not tailored to individual patients. Also, the patient must be able to perform the task of interest and perform it in a timely manner.

Clinical Uses of fMRI

The only clinical use for fMRI that is typically reimbursed is for presurgical planning for tumor resection and epilepsy surgery (Matthews, 2015; Silva, See, Essayed, Golby, & Tie, 2018). There are a variety of uses under investigation that could lead to clinical translation, including determining candidacy for speech and language treatment or treatment method poststroke (Shuster, 2018), and monitoring brain activation during deep brain stimulation in an effort to determine the relationship between patterns of brain activation and therapeutic outcome and/or side effects.

MAGNETIC RESONANCE SPECTROSCOPY

Overview of Magnetic Resonance Spectroscopy

Like fMRI, magnetic resonance spectroscopy (MRS) is performed in the MR scanner.

Whereas MRI and fMRI can provide important information about structure and function, they do not provide information that can be used to differentiate different pathological processes. For example, it can be difficult to distinguish between a cerebral infarction and a glioma using MRI. MRS provides chemical information about tissues (Soares & Law, 2009; Tognarelli et al., 2015). It is also called nuclear magnetic resonance spectroscopy, but the "nuclear" is usually omitted in the name to avoid confusion with nuclear medicine, which was described above in the section on PET (van der Graaf, 2010).

MRS Details

As with MRI, the most common MRS method images hydrogen because of its properties when placed in a magnetic field, as described above in the section on MRI. In addition, it is ubiquitous in different tissues, and the characteristics of the signal it generates when placed in the magnetic field depend on its chemical environment. The chemical environment refers to its location(s) within a molecule. Molecules or metabolites that are important for the function of the central nervous system, such as choline, alanine, and lipids, have different nuclear magnetic resonance signals, as well as different distributions within tissues (Ulmer, Backens, & Ahlhelm, 2016). For example, the presence of lipids reveals information about tissue necrosis and cancer metastases.

MRS techniques may image a single voxel or multiple voxels. Similar to the way in which speech can be displayed acoustically, the MRS data from the voxel or voxels are usually displayed as line spectra. A speech line spectrum reveals the frequencies that are present in the speech signal, and the height of the line represents the intensity of those frequencies.

MRS spectra serve as a fingerprint for identifying the metabolites that are detected in the voxel(s), and the height of the peak represents the relative amount of the metabolite (Ulmer, Backens, & Ahlhelm, 2016).

MRS is subject to the same types of artifact as MRI and fMRI, including artifact induced by head motion. MRS has low SNR and relatively poor spatial resolution (Ratai & Gonzalez, 2016). As with other MRI approaches, SNR improves with increased magnetic field strength, so better SNR is obtained at 3T than at 1.5T. The spatial resolution of single voxel MRS is on the order of 3 to 8 cm^3, whereas for multivoxel MRS, it is 0.5 to 3 cm^3 (Ratai & Gonzalez).

Advantages and Disadvantages of MRS

As noted above, the main advantage of MRS is that it provides information on the biochemistry of tissues, which serves as an important diagnostic adjunct to other neuroimaging methods, such as structural MRI. One disadvantage is that the absolute concentration of the metabolites in a voxel or voxels is not known; therefore, they are calculated as relative values, as noted above (Ulmer, Backens, & Ahlhelm, 2016).

Clinical Uses of MRS

Currently, MRS is typically reimbursed for the study of tumors. For example, Aetna considers MRS medically necessary for tumor-related studies such as distinguishing low-grade from high-grade tumors, determining whether a biopsy or resection can be safely postponed, and distinguishing recurrent brain tumor from radiation-induced necrosis.

DIFFUSION WEIGHTED MAGNETIC RESONANCE IMAGING

Overview of Diffusion Weighted Magnetic Resonance Imaging

Diffusion weighted magnetic resonance imaging (DWI) is the study of the movement of water molecules in the body that is measured in the MRI scanner (Chilla, Tan, Xu, & Poh, 2015; Koh & Collins, 2007). Water molecules, for example in a glass of water, are moving relatively freely in constant random (Brownian) motion. When water can move freely in all directions, it is described as isotropic, that is, there is no preferred direction of movement. However, in human tissue, the movement of water molecules is restricted as a function of tissue type, structure, integrity, and the presence of barriers (Koh & Collins, 2007; Soares, Marques, Alves, & Sousa, 2013). When the direction of movement is restricted, it is described as being anisotropic; the diffusion is not the same in all directions. Think of a group of people standing around in a room. They are free to move around in a variety of directions, that is, their movement is isotropic. However, if you ask those people to move to another room by walking down a narrow hallway, their movement down the hallway is much more restricted, that is, it is anisotropic. The signal that is used to create the DWI maps is a function of the rate of movement of water molecules outside of cells, from the outside to the inside of cells, and within the vasculature. DWI maps represent tissue contrast (Soares et al., 2013).

DWI Details

Diffusion tensor imaging (DTI) is a method for modeling DWI data sets using what are called diffusion tensors (Huisman, 2010; Soares et al., 2013). Anisotropy occurs on a continuum related to the degree to which the diffusion is restricted. If we return to the analogy of people moving down a hallway, movement down a narrow hallway would be more restricted than movement down a wider hallway. Cerebrospinal fluid has a low degree of anisotropy, whereas brain gray matter has a higher degree of anisotropy. White matter has an even higher degree of anisotropy due to the association of parallel axons. The nerve cell's membrane restricts the motion of water in the intracellular fluid in the direction perpendicular to the axon, so that the direction of movement is along the long axis of the axon. Thus, DTI provides a method for studying the integrity of white matter in the brain.

The spatial resolution of DWI is on the order of 2 mm (Chilla et al., 2015). Artifacts arise from the same sources as other types of studies performed in the MRI scanner, especially head motion. However, an additional source of artifact that has been identified in DTI is from the mechanical vibration of the scanner (Berl et al., 2015).

Advantages and Disadvantages of DWI

The advantages of the DWI modalities are that they make use of endogenous contrast, and it provides a method for studying brain connections. A disadvantage of DTI is that the data analysis has been time consuming and data interpretation can be challenging (Huisman, 2010), although the manufacturers of MRI scanners continue to develop methods to streamline the analysis.

Clinical Uses of DWI

DWI is useful for studying tumors, because they have high cell density, which results in more restricted diffusion (Chilla et al., 2015). As a result, DTI is a valuable tool for brain mapping prior to tumor surgery (Ulmer, Klein, Mueller, DeYoe, & Mark, 2014). It is also highly sensitive to ischemic brain infarction (Holdsworth & Bammer, 2008). Another use is for the study of white matter disease, such as multiple sclerosis (Baliyan, Das, Sharma, & Gupta, 2016). Additional clinical uses include imaging arterial dissections, Creutzfeldt-Jakob's disease, and inflammatory disease such as optic neuritis (Drake-Perez, Boto, Fitsiori, Lovblad, & Vargas, 2018). Although DWI has been suggested for other uses, further technical developments and standardization are required before widespread clinical adoption can occur for imaging in areas such as epilepsy, traumatic brain injury, and Alzheimer's disease (Lerner, Mogensen, Kim, Shiroishi, Hwang, & Law, 2014).

ELECTROENCEPHALOGRAPHY

Overview of Electroencephalography

Electroencephalography (EEG) measures electrical signals from the brain using instrumentation that is located outside of the brain. Thus, unlike the more direct approach of recording electrical signals by inserting an electrode into a nerve cell, EEG is noninvasive. EEG is conducted by positioning electrodes on the scalp. These can either be single electrodes, attached to a cap or attached to a net. It is recommended that a minimum of 21 electrodes be used for clinical purposes, although fewer may be used for individuals with smaller heads, such as infants (Tatum, 2014; Tufenkjian, 2017).

EEG Details

Electrical signals in the brain are produced by the movement of electrical charges (current flow), which occurs in neurons during the generation of action potentials (APs), and during the postsynaptic potentials (PSPs) that are induced by the action potentials (Tatum, 2014). During PSPs, electrical current flows within and around the neuron, and the PSPs can be either excitatory (EPSPs), making it more likely that the neuron will generate an action potential, or inhibitory (IPSPs), making it less likely that the neuron will generate an action potential. The source of the signal that is measured in EEG comes mainly from PSPs, which are of longer duration and have larger current than action potentials (Baillet, 2017). This is important, because the signal must have sufficient strength to propagate through meninges, skull, and skin in order to be recorded on the surface of the head. In particular, a main source of the signal recorded in EEG is PSPs of pyramidal neurons in the cerebral cortex, which have several properties that make it possible to record their current from outside of the brain. One property is that the PSPs in pyramidal neurons are of longer duration than APs, which means that the PSPs are more likely to overlap temporally despite not being totally synchronized with one another; thus, the overlap increases the likelihood that the PSPs will sum together and produce a larger signal (Baillet, 2017; Tatum, 2014). The other property of pyramidal neurons is that they are oriented similarly, that is, with their apical dendrites (which is where much of the post-synaptic current flow occurs) perpendicular to the cortical surface. The consistent, similar orientation increases the summation of the currents in space. The postsynaptic current, the primary current, flows across the cell membrane at the synapse and continues intracellularly, whereas a secondary or volume current is generated by the flow of an equivalent current in the extracellular space (Wibral, Bledowski, & Turi, 2010). EEG detects the volume or extracellular current.

The gold standard in EEG is the use of wet electrodes, which involve a somewhat time- and labor-intensive setup process (Lopez-Gordo, Sanchez-Morillo, & Valle, 2014). Wet means that a paste or gel must be applied between the electrode and scalp to facilitate signal transmission. The sites for placement of the electrodes have been standardized using the 10-20 system, which uses anatomical landmarks on the skull to try to ensure consistent placement across patients (Klem, Lüders, Jasper, & Elger, 1999); however, there is individual variability in the size and shape of heads, so this must be taken into account. The outer layer of the skin is a source of electrical resistance that should, ideally, be minimized. Thus, once the sites for electrode placement are determined, they must be scrubbed with an abrasive paste to remove the outer layer of skin. Unfortunately, the gel can be difficult to get out of the hair. If the recording is to occur over a longer time period, the electrodes may be attached to the skull with a compound called collodion (Tatum, 2014). Once the electrodes are in place, the electrode-skin impedance must be tested to ensure that it is low. Although wet electrodes are the gold standard, dry electrodes continue to be developed because they would be simpler to employ (Lopez-Gordo et al., 2014).

A basic EEG signal or channel is the difference in voltage measured between a pair of electrodes. These differences are measured among multiple combinations of electrodes in a systematic way, and the configuration for making these comparisons is referred to as a montage (Tufenkjian, 2017). The signals are amplified and filtered to remove noise, which can arise from the patient or from external sources. The data are then displayed graphically showing the timing and amplitude of the signal recorded from each channel. The SNR of EEG is poor because the signal is so small; thus, it may require averaging many trials in order to detect the signal (Crist & Lebedev, 2008). The spatial resolution of EEG is problematic, primarily because, although the electrodes are placed systematically over the brain, they are located on the scalp and not directly on the brain. As a result, a given signal is simultaneously picked up by many electrodes, not just by the one that is over an area of active cortex. Thus, it is difficult to identify the precise location of the source of the signal detected by a particular electrode, something that is referred to as the inverse problem (Lopez Rincon & Shimoda, 2016). Currently, there is a great deal of research aimed at developing methods for solving the inverse problem, which aims to constrain all of the solutions except the one that best describes the data (Lopes da Silva, 2013). Figure 3–6 shows a photograph of an EEG cap as well as a graph of the EEG signal.

Advantages and Disadvantages of EEG

Unlike the spatial resolution of EEG, the temporal resolution is excellent, which is one of its main advantages. Other advantages are that it provides useful information regarding brain function, regardless of whether the patient is performing a task (unlike fMRI). Thus, it can be used with infants or individuals with altered levels of consciousness. One major disadvantage is that it cannot be used to routinely study speech production or swallowing because the muscle movement involved in those tasks generates large electrical artifacts. Other sources of artifacts can include vascular pulsations, eye blinks, and eye movements, as well as other instrumentation, especially when it is used in environments such as the intensive care unit or the operating room (Puce & Hälämäinen, 2017; Tatum, 2014).

Clinical Uses of EEG

The major clinical use of EEG is in the study of epilepsy. It can help determine the seizure

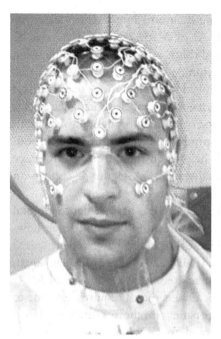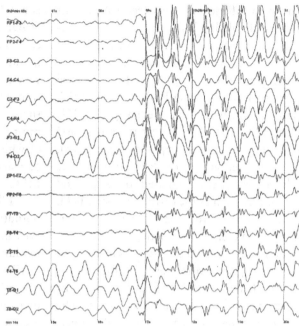

Figure 3–6. Example of an EEG cap, and an EEG graphical recording. Each row in the graph represents the electrical activity recorded from a specific electrode. *Source:* https://commons.wikimedia. org/wiki/File:EEG_cap.jpg. This work has been released into the public domain by its author, Thuglas at English Wikipedia. This applies worldwide. Thuglas grants anyone the right to use this work for any purpose, without any conditions, unless such conditions are required by law. https://en.wikipedia. org/wiki/Spike-and-wave. Uploaded from the German Wikipedia, uploaded into the German Wikipedia by Der Lange 11/6/2005, created by himself. This file is licensed under the Creative Commons Attribution-Share Alike 2.0 Generic license.

type and syndrome which, in turn, guides the selection of antiepileptic medication. It can also help determine prognosis (Smith, 2005).

MAGNETOENCEPHALOGRAPHY

Overview of Magnetoencephalography

Magnetoencephalography (MEG) is a measure of brain function, and, like EEG, it is a more direct measure of neuronal function than PET or fMRI. It is a noninvasive technique that measures magnetic fields generated by neuronal activity in the brain. The sensors

that detect the magnetic fields are housed in a large, helmet-like structure. The strength of the neuronal magnetic fields is very, very small. One analogy is that compared to the magnetic fields generated by an MRI scanner, it is like the sound of a pin being dropped during a rock concert (Proudfoot, Woolrich, Nobre, & Turner, 2014).

MEG Details

As noted above in the discussion of EEG, there are primary and secondary (or volume) electrical currents in PSPs, in addition to those generated by APs. Similar to the magnetic field generated by passing current through a wire in an MRI scanner, the electrical currents that are circulating between and within neurons generate tiny electromagnetic fields, and it is these magnetic fields that are detected in MEG, primarily those produced by electrical currents flowing during PSPs (Baillet, 2017; Hari & Salmelin, 2012; Lopes da Silva, 2013). Thus, EEG and MEG detect the same basic neuronal phenomena (Lopes da Silva, 2013). As mentioned above, these electromagnetic fields are very weak compared to background magnetism, such as the earth's magnetic field. In fact, the electronic devices in a laboratory generate electromagnetic fields that can be as much as a thousand times greater than the fields generated by neurons (Parkkonen, 2010). Therefore, the MEG hardware must be sensitive enough to detect the tiny signal. The only device that has this capacity is the super-conducting quantum interference device, or SQUID. As in MRI, the SQUID must be cooled and this is also accomplished by using liquid helium. In addition, the MEG hardware must be located in a room that shields it from external sources of electromagnetic fields (noise), and equipment brought into the room must not produce electromagnetic noise, both of which help to ensure optimal SNR (Puce & Hälämäinen, 2017). Figure 3–7 shows an MEG scanner.

Like EEG, MEG has excellent temporal resolution at the submillisecond level; however, unlike EEG, it also has excellent spatial resolution (Baillet, 2017; Puce & Hälämäinen, 2017). There are several advantages of MEG over EEG. One is that it requires less time to prepare the patient for the measurement. However, as noted above, there are standard pro-

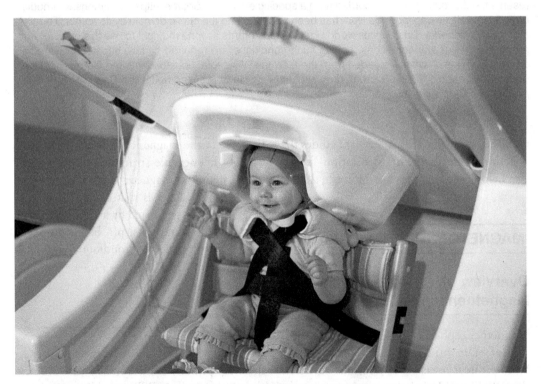

Figure 3–7. Magnetoencephalography scanner. The helmet above the infant's head contains the SQUID sensors and the liquid helium used for cooling the sensors. *Source:* Courtesy of the Institute for Learning and Brain Sciences, University of Washington.

cedures for orienting the electrodes in EEG, whereas in MEG, hardware differences among manufacturers, along with potential differences in patient position within the device, make comparisons across and within patients more challenging (Baillet, 2017). Moreover, the MEG signal is not affected by traveling through the tissues overlaying the brain to the signal detector (Puce & Hälämäinen, 2017). For both EEG and MEG, signals arising from brain regions below the cerebral cortex, such as the hippocampus, are weak and thus can be difficult to detect, but this is more of a problem for MEG than EEG. MEG is most sensitive to currents that are tangential to the scalp, in particular, neurons in the sulci of the cerebral cortex, whereas EEG is sensitive to both tangential currents and radial currents (from neurons in the gyri: Ahlfors, Han, Belliveau, & Hälämäinen, 2010; Baillet, 2017; Lopes da Silva, 2013, Puce & Hälämäinen, 2017). This difference in sensitivity is partly what contributes to the better spatial resolution of MEG.

Advantages and Disadvantages of MEG

Unlike EEG, where moving the jaw and tongue produces artifact, MEG can be used to study speech production (Hari & Salmelin, 2012). Like EEG and unlike fMRI, it does not require the patient to perform a task. In addition to electronic instrumentation in the MEG room, eye movements and blinks can produce artifacts in MEG. Other sources of noise can be problematic, such as vibrations, nearby elevators, and air conditioning units. As with many of the neuroimaging modalities, head motion can be a problem (Puce & Hälämäinen, 2017). A major disadvantage of MEG is its cost. According to megcommunity.org, there are 40 MEG units in the United States, and they are located in large cities and/or academic medical settings (http://megcommunity.org/groups-jobs/groups); thus, they are not accessible for many people, although there are more in the United States than any other country.

Clinical Uses of MEG

The main clinical use for MEG is in the study of epilepsy. For example, it is being used to determine the source of the epileptogenic activity and to identify eloquent cortex for the purpose of surgical planning with both adults and children (Schwartz et al., 2008). This allows the surgical team to evaluate the likelihood of success with regard to eliminating seizures and also to estimate the extent of postsurgical behavioral deficits as a result of resection of the tumor.

NEUROSONOLOGY

Overview of Neurosonology

As the "sono" portion of its name suggests, neurosonology imaging methods employ ultrasound. With regard to neuroimaging, it is used to study the arteries. During diagnostic ultrasound, a transducer is placed on or in the body, such as on the skin. The transducer generates sound waves that travel into the body and then are reflected back to the transducer (Gerhard-Herman, 2005). The strength and timing of the returning sound, or echo, is used to generate an image.

Neurosonology Details

The basic mode employed in neurosonology is called the brightness mode (B-mode; Abu-Zidan, Hefner, & Corr, 2011). This provides two-dimensional black and white imaging. An important use of B-mode ultrasound is for measuring the thickness of the arterial walls of the common carotid arteries for the purpose of diagnosing atherosclerosis (Loizou et al,, 2015).

Doppler ultrasound can be used to study blood flow in the head and neck vasculature, including the middle, anterior and posterior arteries, as well as the carotids. As its name implies, it is based on the principle of the Doppler effect (Kassab et al., 2007; Kirsch, Mathur, Johnson, Gowthaman, & Scoutt, 2013). When a sound wave of a particular frequency encounters red blood cells, the sound is reflected back at a lower or higher frequency. The difference in frequency between what is emitted and what is reflected back to the transducer is known as the Doppler shift, and it can be used to calculate the velocity and direction of the blood flow.

The spatial and contrast resolution in ultrasound are influenced by a variety of factors related to parameters, such as the length and frequency of the acoustic pulse, but the temporal resolution is excellent (Akif Topcuoglu, 2012; Ng & Swanevelder, 2011). Contrast agents can be used to enhance contrast.

Advantages and Disadvantages of Neurosonology

One of the major advantages of neurosonology is that ultrasound is not invasive. It is also portable, has a lower cost than other modalities for imaging the vasculature, such as MRA, and can be used in patients with altered consciousness (Akif Topcuoglu, 2012; Lau & Arntfield, 2017). A disadvantage is that is not a direct measure.

Clinical Uses of Neurosonology

Doppler ultrasound is used for several purposes, including the diagnosis of vasospasm and arterial stenosis. Another important use is for the diagnosis of sickle cell disease, which involves progressive occlusion of the large intracranial arteries (Kassab et al., 2007).

THE FUTURE

Continued improvements in technology to enhance spatial and temporal resolution, provide better ways to address artifacts, and reduce the cost of the technology can be expected, although there may be limits to what can be achieved for the noninvasive imaging of the human brain (Thomas et al., 2014). A major focus of research relates to ways of combining neuroimaging methods in order to take advantage of the strengths of one to make up for the weaknesses of another. For example, combining fMRI with EEG results in imaging that has both excellent spatial resolution and temporal resolution. The biggest challenge is combining technologies that are compatible with one another. If a traditional EEG system is introduced into the environment of the MRI scanner, this presents significant problems, including introducing artifacts in the EEG, and focal burns to the patient due to heating of the electrodes and cables (Hari & Puce, 2017). Thus, MRI-compatible EEG systems were developed and are now available. Combined PET/MRI scanners have been developed, although they have yet to see widespread clinical adoption. MRI images, which provide better spatial localization than CT, can then be registered to the PET scans. In addition, further developments in existing technologies will help improve aspects of imaging, such as spatial resolution. Although EEG as traditionally used is not invasive, a recently developed invasive method called stereoelectroencephalography (SEEG) is being increasingly paired with other imaging techniques to locate epileptogenic foci for the surgical management of epilepsy (Abel, Losito, Ibrahim, Asano, & Rutka, 2018). SEEG involves recording from electrodes implanted directly into the brain.

In addition to new developments in technology, there will be an increase in the different uses of existing neuroimaging technologies as research evidence for the clinical utility of the information continues to mount. However, this increased use must also be supported with high quality evidence regarding the mechanisms underlying human neurogenic disease. As mentioned earlier, PET imaging of beta amyloid for the diagnosis of Alzheimer's disease (AD) is not generally reimbursed because it is still considered investigational. More importantly, the role that beta amyloid plays in the development of AD is controversial (Demetrius, Magistretti, & Pellerin, 2015). Thus, the utility of neuroimaging to improve diagnosis must be subjected to rigorous analysis on a variety of levels. Another potential use of neuroimaging could be to predict outcomes, for example in communication disorders, but this use must also be subjected to rigorous scrutiny (Shuster, 2018). Future clinical use of neuroimaging could involve diagnosis of Parkinson's disease, Huntington's disease, and multiple sclerosis (Politis & Piccini, 2012).

In summary, neuroimaging has revolutionized the diagnosis and treatment of neuropathologies. These technologies can provide important information, however, they also have their weaknesses and limitations, as summarized in Table 3–1. Although it is likely that some of these weaknesses and limitations will be addressed with future developments in both the technology and our understanding of the neuropathologies, they must be used judiciously and will continue to be an adjunct, not a substitute, for good clinical observation and judgment. Importantly, the information presented here is a brief overview of the methods. It is recommended that the reader who is interested in greater detail consult the references listed in the reference list.

CASE STUDIES

Case Study #1

A 7-year-old male was referred to the school speech-language pathologist (SLP) by his teacher for the evaluation of his language skills. The child appeared to have increasing difficulty in understanding what was said to him and had begun to perform more poorly in school. He had undergone a complete audiological evaluation, and his hearing was within normal limits. His Receptive Language Index standard score on the Clinical Evaluation of Language Fundamentals-5 (CELF-5) was 69, which was equivalent to a percentile rank of 2. His Expressive Language Index standard score was also somewhat depressed at 78 (percentile rank of 7). Due to the progressive nature of the problem, the SLP advised the child's parents to ask his pediatrician for a referral to a neurologist. Along with the neurological examination, the neurologist ordered a series of tests. The child's MRI was normal, as was an analysis of his cerebrospinal fluid. Awake EEG was normal, however, he demonstrated electrical status epilepticus of sleep (ESES). ESES is a phenomenon in which frequent spike and slow waves appear at the onset of sleep. This pattern occurs almost continually through most of the nonrapid eye movement sleep cycles. Based on the language symptoms and the EEG pattern, the neurologist diagnosed him with Landau-Kleffner syndrome. The child was placed on antiepileptic drugs and enrolled in speech-language therapy.

Case Study #2

A 68-year-old man with a history of hypertension and hyperlipidemia presented to the emergency department with sudden onset of

Table 3–1. A Comparison of Clinical Neuroimaging Methods

Imaging Method	Structure or Function?	Invasive?	Primary Clinical Uses	Other Information
Computerized Tomography (CT)	Structure	Yes, ionizing radiation	Stroke, tumor	Widely available; typically, the first technique used in suspected stroke; used with and without contrast
Positron Emission Tomography (PET)	Function	Yes, radioactive contrast, ionizing radiation	Tumor, presurgical planning	Limited availability due to need for cyclotron; gold standard for tumor imaging
Magnetic Resonance Imaging (MRI)	Structure	No	Stroke	Almost as widely available as CT; very sensitive to head motion; used with and without contrast; not safe for all patients; machine is noisy
Functional Magnetic Resonance Imaging (fMRI)	Function	No	Presurgical planning	Image processing is complex; very sensitive to head motion; not safe for all patients; indirect measure of neuronal activity
Magnetic Resonance Spectroscopy (MRS)	Function	No	Tumor	Very sensitive to head motion; provides information on tissue biochemistry
Diffusion Weighted Imaging (DWI)	Structure	No	Tumor, white matter disease, arterial dissections, inflammatory disease	Very sensitive to head motion; data processing is time consuming; data interpretation can be challenging
Electro-encephalography (EEG)	Function	No	Epilepsy	Excellent temporal resolution; can be administered in a variety of ways, for example, awake, asleep, during everyday activities; direct measure of neuronal activity
Magneto-encephalography (MEG)	Function	No	Epilepsy	Limited availability; expensive; machine is quiet; direct measure of neuronal activity
Neurosonology	Structure	No	Structure of the arteries	Portable; can be used with patients who have altered consciousness

speech problems and weakness of the right side. On examination, he demonstrated aphasia, left gaze preference, a right visual field cut, right lower face droop, dysarthria, and right hemiplegia. His NIH Stroke Scale (NIHSS) was 19, suggesting a moderate-severe stroke. CT of the head revealed hyperdensity in the M1 segment of the left middle cerebral artery (LMCA) territory, with no other signs suggestive of an ischemic stroke, however, CT angiography revealed occlusion of the LMCA. He was administered intravenous tissue plasminogen activator (tPA) at 1.5 hours after symptom onset. Multimodal MRI completed at 3 hours after symptom onset revealed ischemic changes that were confined predominantly to the LMCA. Perfusion-weighted MRI showed larger perfusion abnormality, indicating presence of a substantial volume of potentially salvageable penumbral tissue. Magnetic resonance angiography showed a loss of signal in the LMCA. Cerebral angiography revealed a thrombus, indicating that the tPA had not been successful in dissolving the clot. As a result, a mechanical thrombectomy (physical retrieval of the clot) was performed at approximately 4.5 hours after symptom onset. The next day, he demonstrated only a mild aphasia and right facial droop, and at three months poststroke, he had no residual deficits.

Case Study #3

A 70-year-old female who presented with gradual onset of language problems and suspected ischemia was referred for neurologic evaluation. CT and MRI revealed a lesion in the left frontoparietal region surrounded by edema, with characteristics that indicated it could be a metastatic lesion. PET was ordered to confirm the presence of the brain lesion and look for a primary tumor. A PET scan using FDG radioactive tracer revealed high glucose uptake in the left frontoparietal region with an adjacent hypometabolic region—a pattern suggestive of a tumor. A hypermetabolic focus was seen in left lateral frontal lobe. Chest and abdominal CT revealed no additional lesions. Surgery revealed a small grade III anaplastic astrocytoma surrounded by edema.

Case Study #4

A 7-year-old boy with a 5-year history of recurrent, uncontrolled seizures of undetermined etiology was referred to a pediatric neurologist. Despite taking a combination of antiepileptic medications at high doses, he continued to experience multiple seizures per day. Previous trials of antiepileptic medications had failed to control his seizures. Although his cognitive and social development appeared to be normal, the seizures had a significant negative effect on quality of life, as did the side effects of the antiepileptic medications. He underwent a 5-day video-electroencephalography (vEEG) evaluation to record and characterize his seizures. The vEEG suggested that the seizures were arising from the left side of the brain, but they were unable to be localized with any further accuracy. MRI of the brain did not reveal any structural abnormalities. Additional noninvasive tests were performed, including ictal SPECT and interictal FDG-PET, but the results also were not helpful in localizing the seizure focus. As a result, he was not considered a candidate for epilepsy surgery.

Three years later, the seizures had continued unabated, and the patient was referred to a pediatric neurologist for reevaluation. MRI with higher spatial resolution was again within normal limits. However, he also underwent MEG, and these results provided more localizing information, which allowed for surgical intervention. His antiepileptic medications were subsequently reduced. Two years postsurgery he was seizure-free and performing well in school.

Case Study #5

A 24-year-old man was referred to a neurologist complaining of intermittent speech arrest. CT revealed a lesion in left frontal lobe with edema surrounding the lesion. Magnetic resonance spectroscopy (MRS) demonstrated mildly depressed N-acetylaspartate (NAA) and elevated choline, and the choline revealed a "hot spot" that was used as a target for a biopsy. He was subsequently scheduled for surgical resection of a grade II astrocytoma. The neurosurgeon and neurologist requested clinical fMRI to localize speech and language with the aim of preserving speech and language function and also to better delineate the area of planned tumor resection. The patient performed two tasks in the scanner, word generation, and verb generation. The neurosurgeon was able to avoid the area that demonstrated activation during the language tasks and 6 months postsurgery, the patient demonstrated no language deficits.

REFERENCES

Abel, T. J., Losito, E., Ibrahim, G. M., Asano, E., & Rutka, J. T. (2018). Multimodal localization and surgery for epileptic spasms of focal origin: a review. *Neurosurgical Focus, 45*(3), E4. https://doi.org/10.3171/2018.6.FOCUS18217

Abu-Zidan, F. M., Hefny, A. F., & Corr, P. (2011). Clinical ultrasound physics. *Journal of Emergencies, Trauma, and Shock, 4*(4), 501–503. https://doi.org/10.4103/0974-2700.86646

Ahlfors, S. P., Han, J., Belliveau, J. W., & Hämäläinen, M. S. (2010). Sensitivity of MEG and EEG to source orientation. *Brain Topography, 23*(3), 227–232. https://doi.org/10.1007/s10548-010-0154-x

Akif Topcuoglu, M. (2012). Transcranial Doppler ultrasound in neurovascular diseases: Diagnostic and therapeutic aspects. *Journal of Neurochemistry, 123*, 39–51. https://doi.org/10.1111/j.1471-4159.2012.07942.x

Alvares, R. D. A., Szulc, D. A., & Cheng, H-L. M. (2017). A scale to measure MRI contrast agent sensitivity. *Scientific Reports, 7*(1), 15493. https://doi.org/10.1038/s41598-017-15732-8

American College of Obstetricians and Gynecologists. (2017). Guidelines for diagnostic imaging during pregnancy and lactation. Committee Opinion No. 723. *Obstetrics and Gynecology, 130*, e210–e216.

Andre, J. B., Bresnahan, B. W., Mossa-Basha, M., Hoff, M. N., Smith, C. P., Anzai, Y., & Cohen, W. A. (2015). Toward quantifying the prevalence, severity, and cost associated with patient motion during clinical MR examinations. *Journal of the American College of Radiology, 12*(7), 689–695. https://doi.org/10.1016/j.jacr.2015.03.007

Antoch, G., Veit, P., Bockisch, A., & Kuehl, H. (2011). Application of CT contrast agents in PET-CT imaging. In P. Shreve & D. W. Townsend (Eds.), *Clinical PET-CT in radiology* (pp. 91–101). New York, NY: Springer. https://doi.org/10.1007/978-0-387-48902-5_9

Baghaei, H., Wong, W-H. G., & Li, H. (2013). Principles of positron emission tomography imaging. In E. E. Kim, M.-C. Lee, T. Inoue, & W.-H. Wong (Eds.), *Clinical PET and PET/CT* (pp. 3–27). New York, NY: Springer. https://doi.org/10.1007/978-1-4419-0802-5_1

Baillet, S. (2017). Magnetoencephalography for brain electrophysiology and imaging. *Nature Neuroscience, 20*(3), 327–339. https://doi.org/10.1038/nn.4504

Baliyan, V., Das, C. J., Sharma, R., & Gupta, A. K. (2016). Diffusion weighted imaging: Technique and applications. *World Journal of Radiology, 8*(9), 785–798. https://doi.org/10.4329/wjr.v8.i9.785

Barrett, J. F., & Keat, N. (2004). Artifacts in CT: Recognition and avoidance. *RadioGraphics, 24*(6), 1679–1691. https://doi.org/10.1148/rg.246045065

Bennett C. M., Baird, A. A., Miller, M. B., & Wolford, G. (2010). Neural correlates of interspecies perspective taking in the post-mortem Atlantic salmon: An argument for proper multiple comparisons correction. *Journal of Serendipitous and Unexpected Results, 1*, 1–5.

Berger, A. (2002). Magnetic resonance imaging. *BMJ (Clinical Research Ed.), 324*(7328), 35. Retrieved from http://www.ncbi.nlm.nih.gov/pubmed/11777806

Berl, M. M., Walker, L., Modi, P., Irfanoglu, M. O., Sarlls, J. E., Nayak, A., & Pierpaoli, C. (2015). Investigation of vibration-induced artifact in clinical diffusion-weighted imaging of pediatric subjects. *Human Brain Mapping, 36*(12), 4745–4757. https://doi.org/10.1002/hbm.22846

Bettinardi, V., Castiglioni, I., De Bernardi, E., & Gilardi, M. C. (2014). PET quantification: Strategies for partial volume correction. *Clinical and Translational Imaging, 2*(3), 199–218. https://doi.org/10.1007/s40336-014-0066-y

Bigler, E. D. (2017). Structural neuroimaging in neuropsychology: History and contemporary applications. *Neuropsychology, 31*(8), 934–953. https://doi.org/10.1037/neu0000418

Birenbaum, D., Bancroft, L. W., & Felsberg, G. J. (2011). Imaging in acute stroke. *Western Journal of Emergency Medicine, 12*(1), 67–76. Retrieved from http://www.ncbi.nlm.nih.gov/pubmed/21694755

Bottinor, W., Polkampally, P., & Jovin, I. (2013). Adverse reactions to iodinated contrast media. *International Journal of Angiology, 22*(3), 149–154.

Brenner, D. J., & Hall, E. J. (2007). Computed tomography—An increasing source of radiation exposure. *New England Journal of Medicine, 357*(22), 2277–2284. https://doi.org/10.1056/NEJMra072149

Buchbinder, B. R. (2016). Functional magnetic resonance imaging. In J. S. Masdeu & R. G. González (Eds.), *Handbook of clinical neurology: Neuroimaging, part I* (Vol. 135, pp. 61–92). Cambridge, MA: Elsevier.

Caldemeyer, K. S., & Buckwalter, K. A. (1999). The basic principles of computed tomography and magnetic resonance imaging. *Journal of the American Academy of Dermatology, 41*(5), 768–771. https://doi.org/10.1016/S0190-9622(99)70015-0

Cendes, F., Theodore, W. H., Brinkmann, B. H., Sulc, V., & Cascino, G. D. (2016). Neuroimaging of epilepsy. In J. C. Masdeu & R. G. González (Eds.), *Handbook of clinical neurology: Neuroimaging, part II* (Vol. 136, pp. 985–1014). https://doi.org/10.1016/B978-0-444-53486-6.00051-X

Chilla, G. S., Tan, C. H., Xu, C., & Poh, C. L. (2015). Diffusion weighted magnetic resonance imaging and its recent trend—a survey. *Quantitative Imaging in Medicine and Surgery, 5*(3), 407–422. https://doi.org/10.3978/j.issn.2223-4292.2015.03.01

Cierniak, R. (2011a). The physics of data acquisition. In *X-Ray computed tomography in biomedical engineering* (pp. 63–81). London, UK: Springer. https://doi.org/10.1007/978-0-85729-027-4_4

Cierniak, R. (2011b). Technical concepts of X-ray computed tomography scanners. In *X-ray computed tomography in biomedical engineering* (pp. 21–62). London, UK: Springer. https://doi.org/10.1007/978-0-85729-027-4_3

Crist, R. E., & Lebedev, M. A. (2008). Multielectrode recording in behaving monkeys. In M. A. L. Nicolelis (Ed.), *Frontiers in neuroscience: Methods for neural ensemble recordings* (pp. 169–188). Boca Raton, FL: CRC Press/Taylor & Francis. Retrieved from http://www.ncbi.nlm.nih.gov/pubmed/21204441

Cronin, C. G., Prakash, P., & Blake, M. A. (2010). Oral and IV contrast agents for the CT portion of PET/CT. *American Journal of Roentgenology, 195*(1), W5–W13. https://doi.org/10.2214/AJR.09.3844

Dale, B. M., Brown, M. A., & Semelka, R. C. (2015). *MRI basic principles and applications*. Chichester, UK: John Wiley & Sons. https://doi.org/10.1002/9781119013068

Demetrius, L. A., Magistretti, P. J., & Pellerin, L. (2015). Alzheimer's disease: The amyloid hypothesis and the Inverse Warburg effect. *Frontiers in Physiology, 5*, 522. https://doi.org/10.3389/fphys.2014.00522

Diba, K., Amarasingham, A., Mizuseki, K., & Buzsáki, G. (2014). Millisecond timescale synchrony among hippocampal neurons. *Journal of Neuroscience, 34*(45), 14984–14994. https://doi.org/10.1523/JNEUROSCI.1091-14.2014

Dorn, F., Liebig, T., Muenzel, D., Meier, R., Poppert, H., Rummeny, E. J., & Huber, A. (2012).

Order of CT stroke protocol (CTA before or after CTP): Impact on image quality. *Neuroradiology, 54*(2), 105–112. https://doi.org/10.1007/s00234-011-0840-8

Drake-Perez, M., Boto, J., Fitsiori, A., Lovblad, K., & Vargas, M.I. (2018). Clinical applications of diffusion weighted imaging in neuroradiology. *Insights into Imaging, 9*, 535–547. https://doi.org/10.1007/s13244-018-0624-3

Ehman, E. C., Johnson, G. B., Villanueva-Meyer, J. E., Cha, S., Leynes, A. P., Larson, P. E. Z., & Hope, T. A. (2017). PET/MRI: Where might it replace PET/CT? *Journal of Magnetic Resonance Imaging, 46*(5), 1247–1262. https://doi.org/10.1002/jmri.25711

Essig, M., Shiroishi, M. S., Nguyen, T. B., Saake, M., Provenzale, J. M., Enterline, D., . . . Law, M. (2013). Perfusion MRI: The five most frequently asked technical questions. *AJR American Journal of Roentgenology, 200*(1), 24–34. https://doi.org/10.2214/AJR.12.9543

Ezzeddine, M. A., Lev, M. H., McDonald, C. T., Rordorf, G., Oliveira-Filho, J., Aksoy, F. G., . . . Koroshetz, W. J. (2002). CT angiography with whole brain perfused blood volume imaging: Added clinical value in the assessment of acute stroke. *Stroke, 33*(4), 959–966. https://doi.org/10.1161/HS0402.105388

Fink, J. R., Muzi, M., Peck, M., & Krohn, K. A. (2015). Multimodality brain tumor imaging: MR imaging, PET, and PET/MR imaging. *Journal of Nuclear Medicine, 56*(10), 1554–1561. https://doi.org/10.2967/jnumed.113.131516

Food and Drug Administration (2018). *Pediatric x-ray imaging*. Retrieved from https://www.fda.gov/Radiation-EmittingProducts/RadiationEmittingProductsandProcedures/MedicalImaging/ucm298899.htm

Gerard, C. S., Tan, L. A., McKhann, G. M., & Byrne, R. W. (2016). Epilepsy surgery in eloquent cortex. In R.W. Byrne (Ed.), *Functional mapping of the cerebral cortex* (pp. 171–179). Switzerland: Springer. https://doi.org/10.1007/978-3-319-23383-3_11

Gerhard-Herman, M. (2005). Principles of vascular laboratory testing. In E. R. Mohler, M. Gerhard-Herman, & M. R. Jaff (Eds.), *Essentials of vascular laboratory diagnosis* (pp. 3–11). Malden, MA: Blackwell.

Griffeth, L. K. (2005). Use of PET/CT scanning in cancer patients: Technical and practical considerations. *Proceedings (Baylor University. Medical Center), 18*(4), 321–330. Retrieved from http://www.ncbi.nlm.nih.gov/pubmed/16252023

Gulani, V., Calamante, F., Shellock, F. G., Kanal, E., Reeder, S. B., & International Society for Magnetic Resonance in Medicine. (2017). Gadolinium deposition in the brain: Summary of evidence and recommendations. *The Lancet. Neurology, 16*(7), 564–570. https://doi.org/10.1016/S1474-4422(17)30158-8

Hao, X., Xu, D., Bansal, R., Dong, Z., Liu, J., Wang, Z., . . . Peterson, B. S. (2013). Multimodal magnetic resonance imaging: The coordinated use of multiple, mutually informative probes to understand brain structure and function. *Human Brain Mapping, 34*(2), 253–271. https://doi.org/10.1002/hbm.21440

Hari, R., & Puce, A. (2017). *MEG-EEG primer*. New York, NY: Oxford University Press.

Hari, R., & Salmelin, R. (2012). Magnetoencephalography: From SQUIDs to neuroscience: Neuroimage 20th Anniversary Special Edition. *NeuroImage, 61*(2), 386–396. https://doi.org/10.1016/J.NEUROIMAGE.2011.11.074

Hartung, M. P., Grist, T. M., & François, C. J. (2011). Magnetic resonance angiography: Current status and future directions. *Journal of Cardiovascular Magnetic Resonance, 13*(1), 19. https://doi.org/10.1186/1532-429X-13-19

Havsteen, I., Ohlhues, A., Madsen, K. H., Nybing, J. D., Christensen, H., & Christensen, A. (2017). Are movement artifacts in magnetic resonance imaging a real problem?—A narrative review. *Frontiers in Neurology, 8*, 232. https://doi.org/10.3389/fneur.2017.00232

Holdsworth, S. J., & Bammer, R. (2008). Magnetic resonance imaging techniques: fMRI, DWI, and PWI. *Seminars in Neurology, 28*(4), 395–406. https://doi.org/10.1055/s-0028-1083697

Huisman, T. A. G. M. (2010). Diffusion-weighted and diffusion tensor imaging of the brain, made easy. *Cancer Imaging, 10*(1A), S163–S171. https://doi.org/10.1102/1470-7330.2010.9023

Kamalian, S. Lev, M. H., & Gupta, R. (2016). Computed tomography imaging and angiograpy—principles. In J. S. Masdeu & R. G.

González (Eds.), *Handbook of clinical neurology: Neuroimaging, part I* (Vol. 135, pp. 3–20). Cambridge, MA: Elsevier.

Karaman, E., Isilkad, H., Yilmaz, M., Enver, O., & Albavram, S. (2011). Encephalomalacia in the frontal lobe: Complication of the endoscopic sinus surgery. *Journal of Craniofacial Surgery, 22*(6), 2374–2375.

Kassab, M. Y., Majid, A., Farooq, M. U., Azhary, H., Hershey, L. A., Bednarczyk, E. M., . . . Johnson, M. D. (2007). Transcranial Doppler: An introduction for primary care physicians. *Journal of the American Board of Family Medicine, 20*(1), 65–71. https://doi.org/10.3122/jabfm.2007.01.060128

Kawaguchi, M., Tateishi, U., Inoue, T., & Kim, E. E. (2013). Artifacts in FDG PET and PET/CT. In E. E. Kim, M.-C. Lee, T. Inoue, & W.-H. Wong (Eds.), *Clinical PET and PET/CT* (pp. 107–119). New York, NY: Springer New York. https://doi.org/10.1007/978-1-4419-0802-5_3

Kim, J. J., & Mukherjee, P. (2013). Static anatomic techniques. In T. P. Naidich, M. Castillo, S. Cha, & J. Smirniotopoulos (Eds.), *Imaging the brain* (pp. 3–22). Philadelphia, PA: Elsevier Saunders.

Kirsch, J. D., Mathur, M., Johnson, M. H., Gowthaman, G., & Scoutt, L. M. (2013). Advances in transcranial Doppler US: Imaging ahead. *RadioGraphics, 33*(1), E1–E14. https://doi.org/10.1148/rg.331125071

Klem, G. H., Lüders, H. O., Jasper, H. H., & Elger, C. (1999). The ten-twenty electrode system of the International Federation. The International Federation of Clinical Neurophysiology. *Electroencephalography and Clinical Neurophysiology. Supplement, 52*, 3–6. Retrieved from http://www.ncbi.nlm.nih.gov/pubmed/10590970

Koh, D.-M., & Collins, D. J. (2007). Diffusion-weighted MRI in the body: Applications and challenges in oncology. *American Journal of Roentgenology, 188*(6), 1622–1635. https://doi.org/10.2214/AJR.06.1403

Lameka, K., Farwell, M. D., & Ichise, M. (2016). Positron emission tomography. In J. S. Masdeu & R. G. González (Eds.), *Handbook of clinical neurology: Neuroimaging, part I* (Vol. 135, pp. 209–228). Cambridge, MA: Elsevier.

Lau, V. I., & Arntfield, R. T. (2017). Point-of-care transcranial Doppler by intensivists. *Critical Ultrasound Journal, 9*(1), 21. https://doi.org/10.1186/s13089-017-0077-9

Lerner, A., Mogensen, M. A., Kim, P. E., Shiroishi, M. S., Hwang, D. H., & Law, M. (2014). Clinical applications of diffusion tensor imaging. *World Neurosurgery, 82*(1–2), 96–109. https://doi.org/10.1016/j.wneu.2013.07.083

Liguori, C., Frauenfelder, G., Massaroni, C., Saccomandi, P., Giurazza, F., Pitocco, F., . . . Schena, E. (2015). Emerging clinical applications of computed tomography. *Medical Devices (Auckland, N.Z.), 8*, 265–278. https://doi.org/10.2147/MDER.S70630

Lin, E. C. (2010). Radiation risk from medical imaging. *Mayo Clinic Proceedings, 85*(12), 1142–1146. https://doi.org/10.4065/mcp.2010.0260

Loizou, C. P., Nicolaides, A., Kyriacou, E., Georghiou, N., Griffin, M., & Pattichis, C. S. (2015). A comparison of ultrasound intima-media thickness measurements of the left and right common carotid artery. *IEEE Journal of Translational Engineering in Health and Medicine, 3*, 1900410. https://doi.org/10.1109/JTEHM.2015.2450735

Lopes da Silva, F. (2013). EEG and MEG: Relevance to neuroscience. *Neuron, 80*(5), 1112–1128. https://doi.org/10.1016/J.NEURON.2013.10.017

Lopez-Gordo, M. A., Sanchez-Morillo, D., & Pelayo Valle, F. (2014). Dry EEG electrodes. *Sensors (Basel, Switzerland), 14*(7), 12847–12870. https://doi.org/10.3390/s140712847

Lopez Rincon, A., & Shimoda, S. (2016). The inverse problem in electroencephalography using the bidomain model of electrical activity. *Journal of Neuroscience Methods, 274*, 94–105. https://doi.org/10.1016/J.JNEUMETH.2016.09.011

Mair, G., & Wardlaw, J. M. (2014). Imaging of acute stroke prior to treatment: current practice and evolving techniques. *British Journal of Radiology, 87*(1040), 20140216. https://doi.org/10.1259/bjr.20140216

Maris, T. G. (2016). Basic quality control in routine MRI. *Physica Medica, 32*, 171. https://doi.org/10.1016/J.EJMP.2016.07.268

Matthews, P. M. (2015). *Clinical applications of fMRI* (pp. 611–632). Boston, MA: Springer. https://doi.org/10.1007/978-1-4899-7591-1_21

Mawlawi, O., Wendt, R., & Wong, W.-H. G. (2013). From PET to PET/CT. In E. E. Kim, M.-C. Lee, T. Inoue, & W.-H. Wong (Eds.), *Clinical PET and PET/CT* (pp. 41–57). New York, NY: Springer. https://doi.org/10.1007/978-1-4419-0802-5_3

Morelli, J. N., Runge, V. M., Ai, F., Attenberger, U., Vu, L., Schmeets, S. H., . . . Kirsch, J. E. (2011). An image-based approach to understanding the physics of MR artifacts. *Radio-Graphics*, *31*(3), 849–866. https://doi.org/10.1148/rg.313105115

Muehllehner, G., & Karp, J. S. (2006). Positron emission tomography. *Physics in Medicine and Biology*, *51*(13), R117–R137. https://doi.org/10.1088/0031-9155/51/13/R08

Munich, S. A., Shakir, H. J., & Snyder, K. V. (2016). Role of CT perfusion in acute stroke management. *Cor et Vasa*, *58*(2), e215–e224. https://doi.org/10.1016/J.CRVASA.2016.01.008

Ng, A., & Swanevelder, J. (2011). Resolution in ultrasound imaging. *Continuing Education in Anaesthesia Critical Care & Pain*, *11*(5), 186–192. https://doi.org/10.1093/bjaceaccp/mkr030

Nichols, T. E. (2012). Multiple testing corrections, nonparametric methods, and random field theory. *NeuroImage*, *62*(2), 811–815. https://doi.org/10.1016/J.NEUROIMAGE.2012.04.014

Overweg, J. (2006) *MRI main field magnets*. Paper presented at the 2006 Annual Meeting of International Society for Magnetic Resonance in Medicine. Retrieved from https://afni.nimh.nih.gov/sscc/staff/rwcox/ISMRM_2006/ISMRM%20M-F%202006/files/TuA_08.pdf

Papanicolaou, A. C. (2017). Overview of basic concepts. In A. C. Papanicolaou (Ed.), *The Oxford handbook of functional brain imaging in neuropsychology and cognitive neurosciences* (pp. 3–12). New York, NY: Oxford University Press.

Parizel, P. M., van den Hauwe, L., De Belder, F., Van Goethem, J., Venstermans, C., Salgado, R., . . . Van Hecke, W. (2010). Magnetic resonance imaging of the brain. In P. Reimer, P. M. Parizel, J. F. M. Meaney, & F. A. Stichnoth (Eds.), *Clinical MR imaging* (pp. 107–195). Berlin,

Heidelberg: Springer. https://doi.org/10.1007/978-3-540-74504-4_2

Parkkonen, L. (2010). Instrumentation and data processing. In P. C. Hansen, M. L. Kringelback, & R. Salmelin (Eds.), *MEG: An introduction to the methods* (pp. 24–64). New York, NY: Oxford University Press.

Passingham, R. E., & Rowe, J. B. (2016). *A short guide to brain imaging: The neuroscience of human cognition*. Oxford, UK: Oxford University Press.

Perrin, V. (2013). *MRI techniques*. Hoboken, NJ: John Wiley & Sons. https://doi.org/10.1002/9781118761281

Politis, M., & Piccini, P. (2012). Positron emission tomography imaging in neurological disorders. *Journal of Neurology*, *259*(9), 1769–1780. https://doi.org/10.1007/s00415-012-6428-3

Pooley, R. A. (2005). Fundamental physics of MR imaging. *RadioGraphics*, *25*(4), 1087–1099. https://doi.org/10.1148/rg.254055027

Powers, W. J., Rabinstein, A. A., Ackerson, T., Adeoye, O. M., Bambakidis, N. C., Becker, K., . . . Tirschwell, D. L. (2018). 2018 Guidelines for the early management of patients with acute ischemic stroke: A guideline for healthcare professionals from the American Heart Association/American Stroke Association. *Stroke*, *49*(3), e46-e99. https://doi.org/10.1161/STR.0000000000000158

Proudfoot, M., Woolrich, M. W., Nobre, A. C., & Turner, M. R. (2014). Magnetoencephalography. *Practical Neurology*, *14*(5), 336–343. https://doi.org/10.1136/practneurol-2013-000768

Puce, A., & Hämäläinen, M. S. (2017). A review of issues related to data acquisition and analysis in EEG/MEG Studies. *Brain Sciences*, *7*(6). https://doi.org/10.3390/brainsci7060058

Ratai, E.-M., & González, R.G. (2016). Clinical magnetic resonance spectroscopy of the central nervous system. In J. S. Masdeu & R. G. González (Eds.), *Handbook of clinical neurology: Neuroimaging, part I* (Vol. 135, pp. 61–92). Cambridge, MA: Elsevier.

Ray, J. G., Vermeulen, M. J., Bharatha, A., Montanera, W. J., & Park, A. L. (2016). Association between MRI exposure during pregnancy and fetal and childhood outcomes. *JAMA*, *316*(9), 952. https://doi.org/10.1001/jama.2016.12126

Rogosnitzky, M., & Branch, S. (2016). Gadolinium-based contrast agent toxicity: A review of known and proposed mechanisms. *Biometals, 29*(3), 365–376. https://doi.org/10.1007/s10534-016-9931-7

Schwartz, E. S., Dlugos, D. J., Storm, P. B., Dell, J., Magee, R., Flynn, T. P., . . . Roberts, T. P. L. (2008). Magnetoencephalography for pediatric epilepsy: How we do it. *American Journal of Neuroradiology, 29*(5), 832–837. https://doi.org/10.3174/ajnr.A1029

Shuster, L. (2018). Considerations for the use of neuroimaging technologies for predicting recovery of speech and language in aphasia. *American Journal of Speech-Language Pathology, 27*, 291–305.

Silva, M. A., See, A. P., Essayed, W. I., Golby, A. J., & Tie, Y. (2018). Challenges and techniques for presurgical brain mapping with functional MRI. *NeuroImage: Clinical, 17*, 794–803. https://doi.org/10.1016/J.NICL.2017.12.008

Smith, S. J. M. (2005). EEG in the diagnosis, classification, and management of patients with epilepsy. *Journal of Neurology, Neurosurgery, and Psychiatry, 76*(Suppl. 2), ii2–ii7. https://doi.org/10.1136/jnnp.2005.069245

Soares, D. P., & Law, M. (2009). Magnetic resonance spectroscopy of the brain: Review of metabolites and clinical applications. *Clinical Radiology, 64*(1), 12–21. https://doi.org/10.1016/j.crad.2008.07.002

Soares, J. M., Marques, P., Alves, V., & Sousa, N. (2013). A hitchhiker's guide to diffusion tensor imaging. *Frontiers in Neuroscience, 7*, 31. https://doi.org/10.3389/fnins.2013.00031

Tatum, W. O. (2014). *Handbook of EEG interpretation*. New York, NY: Demos Medical.

Thomas, C., Ye, F. Q., Irfanoglu, M. O., Modi, P., Saleem, K. S., Leopold, D. A., & Pierpaoli, C. (2014). Anatomical accuracy of brain connections derived from diffusion MRI tractography is inherently limited. *Proceedings of the National Academy of Sciences, 111*(46), 16574–16579. https://doi.org/10.1073/pnas.1405672111

Tognarelli, J. M., Dawood, M., Shariff, M. I. F., Grover, V. P. B., Crossey, M. M. E., Cox, I. J., . . . McPhail, M. J. W. (2015). Magnetic resonance spectroscopy: Principles and techniques: Lessons for clinicians. *Journal of Clinical and Experimental Hepatology, 5*(4), 320–328. https://doi.org/10.1016/j.jceh.2015.10.006

Tufenkjian, K. (2017). EEG instrumentation, montage, polarity, and localization. In M. Z. Koubeissi & N. J. Azar (Eds.), *Epilepsy board review* (pp. 15–32). New York, NY: Springer-Verlag.

Turkington, T. G. (2011). PET imaging basics. In P. Shreve & D. W. Townsend (Eds.), *Clinical PET-CT in radiology: Integrated imaging in oncology* (pp. 21–28). New York, NY: Springer-Verlag.

Ulmer, S., Backens, M., & Ahlhelm, F. J. (2016). Basic principles and clinical applications of magnetic resonance spectroscopy in neuroradiology. *Journal of Computer Assisted Tomography, 40*(1), 1–13. https://doi.org/10.1097/RCT.0000000000000322

Ulmer, J. L., Klein, A. P., Mueller, W. M., DeYoe, E. A., & Mark, L. P. (2014). Preoperative diffusion tensor imaging: Improving neurosurgical outcomes in brain tumor patients. *Neuroimaging Clinics of North America, 24*, 599–617. https://doi.org/10.1016/j.nic.2014.08.002

van der Graaf, M. (2010). In vivo magnetic resonance spectroscopy: Basic methodology and clinical applications. *European Biophysics Journal, 39*(4), 527–540. https://doi.org/10.1007/s00249-009-0517-y

Ward, N. S. (2015a). Does neuroimaging help to deliver better recovery of movement after stroke? *Current Opinion in Neurology, 28*(4), 323–329. https://doi.org/10.1097/WCO.0000000000000223

Ward, N. S. (2015b). Using oscillations to understand recovery after stroke. *Brain, 138*(10), 2811–2813. https://doi.org/10.1093/brain/awv265

Welvaert, M., & Rosseel, Y. (2013). On the definition of signal-to-noise ratio and contrast-to-noise ratio for fMRI data. *PLoS ONE, 8*(11), e77089. https://doi.org/10.1371/journal.pone.0077089

Wibral, M., Bledowski, C., & Turi, G. (2010). Integration of separately recorded EEG/MEG and fMRI data. In M. Ullsperger, & S. Debener (Eds.), *Simultaneous EEG and fMRI: Recording, analysis, and application* (pp. 209–234). New York, NY: Oxford University Press.

Workman, R. B., & Coleman, R. E. (2006). Fundamentals of PET and PET/CT imaging. In R. B. Workman & R. E. Coleman (Eds.), *PET/CT* (pp. 1–22). New York, NY: Springer.

Yousem, D. M. (2014). The economics of functional magnetic resonance imaging: Clinical and research. *Neuroimaging Clinics of North America*, 24, 717–724.

Zani, A., Biella, G., & Proverbio, A. (2012). *Brain imaging techniques: Invasiveness and spa-tial and temporal resolution.* Retrieved from https://erplabcnr.wordpress.com/the-lab/publications/books-book-chapters/book-chapters/

Zhu, A., Lee, D., & Shim, H. (2011). Metabolic positron emission tomography imaging in cancer detection and therapy response. *Seminars in Oncology*, *38*(1), 55–69. https://doi.org/10.1053/j.seminoncol.2010.11.012

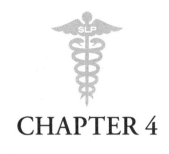

CHAPTER 4

Clinical Considerations of Medication Use in Patients With Swallowing and Communication Disorders

Angela M. Hill, Katlynd Marie Sunjic, Alexandra E. Brandimore,
and Sheeba Varghese Gupta

INTRODUCTION AND RELEVANCE

Medications are not typically a part of the therapeutic interventions for speech-language pathologists; however, their impact on the outcome of speech therapy interventions can be significant. Speech-language pathologists should be able to ascertain the contribution of medication side effects and pharmacological mechanisms to best assist their patients. Older individuals, and those with neurological disorders, such as cerebrovascular disease, Parkinson's disease, and multiple sclerosis, have an increased likelihood of swallowing and communication difficulties, and the use of medications to address these disorders may compound these issues. Medications can be involved in the cause, treatment, and prevention of swallowing disorders. Although medications do not affect communication disorders

directly, their side effects, such as cognitive impairment, sedation, and confusion, can be significant enough to warrant concern. Additionally, although the exact prevalence is unknown, it is estimated that up to 60% of patients may have difficulty swallowing medications, which can negatively impact adherence and therapeutic outcomes (Kelly & Wright, 2009). This difficulty is often under-reported by patients and caregivers, but it is commonly noted in ambulatory, hospitalized, institutionalized, and elderly patients. Thus, it is in the best interest of the speech-language pathologist to have a heightened awareness of issues that will influence medication adherence, as well as the effects of medications on their patients. This chapter discusses how medications are processed by the body and how they impact swallowing or communication. Additionally, key considerations regarding medication use are provided for clinicians to consider when evaluating patients.

Pharmacological Mechanisms Associated With Medications

Pharmacokinetics is the term used to describe the time course, and ultimately the fate, of a medication in the body. Simply put, it is the effect of the body on the medication, and is commonly divided into absorption, distribution, metabolism, and elimination (Williams, 1972).

Absorption

In order for medications to provide their therapeutic effects, they must undergo absorption, distribution into body tissues, and sometimes biotransformation to active metabolites, all which facilitate the medications' effect on the body. The formulation (for example, tablets, capsules, regular, or delayed release formulations) and route of administration of the medication determines the processes by which the medication is able to be absorbed into the blood stream and travel to the desired site of action. The stomach and small intestines allow for most oral dosage formulations of medications to be absorbed, but the cheeks or buccal area, and under the tongue, are alternative oral routes. Medications that are administered by inhalation utilize the lungs for absorption into the body, and this is often the desired site of action as well. Topically administered medications utilize the skin and even the rectum for absorption. As the body ages, the thickness of the skin and other mucosal surfaces may decrease, making medication absorption easier and resulting in increased absorption of topically administered medications (Mangoni & Jackson, 2003).

Distribution

Once the medication is in the blood stream, the body distributes medications into tissues by various mechanisms, utilizing proteins in the blood, such as albumin, to bind and carry the active medication. The amount of medication that reaches the blood, and is not bound to blood proteins, provides the therapeutic effect. Therefore, in patients with hypoalbuminemia (malnourished patients, the elderly population, the acutely ill patient), there may be higher concentrations of medication able to produce a therapeutic effect than in patients without hypoalbuminemia (Mangoni & Jackson, 2003). This increase in medication concentration is often quickly balanced by the body by increasing the clearance of the medication, and therefore the clinical relevance of hypoalbuminemia is variable (Benet & Hoener, 2002). Other factors that impact distribution of medication into tissues include cardiac function, vascular permeability, blood flow, and tissue perfusion rate.

Metabolism

The liver is responsible for biotransforming the medication to its active metabolites, and for metabolizing or breaking down the medication into inactive components. There are enzyme systems in the liver that chemically modify medications so that they are more water soluble, which allows for elimination of medication from the body through bodily fluids, such as the urine. When the liver is diseased, metabolism of medications will be impacted negatively. Also, depending on the patient's age and ethnicity, medications may be metabolized at a slower or faster rate, because of polymorphisms in the various enzyme systems. Lastly, certain medications can "speed up" the liver resulting in a shorter duration of therapeutic effects or "slow down" the metabolic processes of the liver resulting in a longer duration of therapeutic effects or toxicity from certain medications (Alomar, 2014; Wilkinson, 2005).

Elimination

The kidney is also involved in the elimination of medications by various filtration processes. As the body ages, the efficiency of the liver and kidney declines, and may be further compromised by comorbid disease states, such as cirrhosis, diabetes, and heart failure, with reduced left ventricular ejection fraction (Alomar, 2014).

Pharmacodynamics

Pharmacodynamics is the effect that medications have on the body, specifically the physiologic and biochemical effects of the medication (Sera & McPherson, 2012). How a medication exerts these effects is based upon the number and affinity of receptors for the medication at the site of action, the transduction of the signals produced by the interaction of the medication with the receptor, and the body's process for regulation of homeostasis (Turnheim, 1998). How quickly and effectively a medication is absorbed and distributed to the site of action determines its onset of action and affects the timing of the medication's peak, or maximum, effects. This may become clinically significant for medications used in patients with Parkinson's disease, for example, as timing of activities of daily living would ideally be timed when the medication is at its peak effect. As this peak effect differs for all medications, and a complex interplay of pharmacokinetics and pharmacodynamics exists, it is best to locate the pharmacodynamics information in medication information resources or medication package inserts and interpret this information in light of the patient's daily life scenario.

Pharmacological Effects of Medications

Medications demonstrate their effects through neurotransmitter and receptor-mediated processes on organs, glands, and muscles in the sympathetic and parasympathetic systems, resulting in varying therapeutic and side effects. Neurotransmitters are chemicals that facilitate communications between cells. The effects of neurotransmission vary in intensity, depending on factors such as a patient's age, ethnicity, organ function, and medication dose and formulation. Medications are categorized into classes by their pharmacological effects on various receptor subtypes. Table 4–1 describes the primary neurotransmitters and their physiological functions. Neurotransmitters like acetylcholine, serotonin, and glutamate are considered excitatory, whereas gamma aminobutyric acids and dopamine are inhibitory. The neurotransmitters can express excitation or inhibition differently in different parts of the body. For example, serotonin is inhibitory in the spinal cord, but excitatory in the brain. The inhibition of serotonin in the spinal cord assists in the resolution of pain, whereas the excitation of serotonin in the brain alleviates depression and anxiety.

Stimulation, blockade or antagonism, inhibition of reuptake, and other complex pharmacological effects on receptors result in varying responses that are described in Table 4–2. Patients experience these pharmacological effects as therapeutic effects or side effects.

DYSPHAGIA

In elderly patients over 65 years of age, dysphagia affects 7% to 13% (Roy, Stemple, Merrill, & Thomas, 2007). The incidence of dysphagia significantly increases in patients with stroke, postoperative cognitive dysfunction, Parkinson's disease and dementia (Perry, 2001; Setacci et al., 2015). Aging individuals are often susceptible to swallowing difficulties because of the number of medications they use, the number of comorbid problems they are prone to, a decline in organ function affecting the metabolism of medications, and other individual factors (Hajjar, Cafiero, &

Table 4–1. Neurotransmitters, Function, and Receptor Activities

Neurotransmitter	Location of Receptor	Receptor Subtypes	Physiological Function
Acetylcholine	Neuromuscular junction, CNS	Nicotinic Muscarinic	Regulates muscle movement, memory processes
Norepinephrine	Cardiac muscle, adrenal gland, medulla	Adrenergic (α1, α2, β1, β2, β3)	Regulates alertness and arousal
Epinephrine	Cardiac muscle and lungs	Adrenergic (α1, α2, β1, β2, β3)	Regulates cardiovascular and vascular function
Dopamine	Brain, hypothalamus	D1, D2, D3, D4, D5, D7	Regulates appetite, pleasure, and movement
Serotonin	Gut, CNS	5HT1A, 5HT1B, 5HT3, 5HT4, 5HT7	Regulates sleep, appetite, mood, and dilation of vasculature
Histamine	Stomach, brain, smooth muscle	H1, H2, H3, H4	Regulates wound healing, inflammatory responses, promotes wakefulness, regulates appetite, regulates cognition, and mediates itching
Glutamate	CNS, PNS	NMDA and others	Excitatory transmitter that is a precursor to GABA that is key in neural communication, memory formation, learning and regulation
Gamma Amino Butyric Acid (GABA)	CNS	$GABA_A$, $GABA_B$	Primary inhibitory neurotransmitter that is essential in regulation of muscle tone and regulation of anxiety, sleep, and seizures

Sources: Adapted from Brenner & Stevens, 2006; Tiwari, Dwivedi, Singh, Mishra, & Changy, 2017; Li & Xu, 2008; Marieb, 2001; Berger, Gray, & Roth, 2009; Nieto-Alamilla, Marquez-Gomez, Garcia-Galvez, Morales-Figueroa, & Arias-Montano, 2016; Swanson, 2014; Meldrum, 2000; Monoghan, Bridges, & Cotman, 1989; Richelson & Souder, 2000.

Hanlon, 2007). Physiologic changes that occur in the elderly and can cause dysphagia include decreased facial strength, masticatory strength, and lingual pressure; delayed pharyngeal swallow; and atrophy of the pharyngeal musculature (Hara et al., 2018; Molfenter, Brates, Herzberg, Noorani, & Lazarus, 2018). Neurological disorders, gastrointestinal disorders, polypharmacy, autoimmune disorders, traumatic brain injury, and other medical disorders are also associated with causing dysphagia in aging individuals.

Table 4–2. Clinical Issues Related to Neurotransmitter Functioning

Neurotransmitter	Clinical Consequence of Receptor Stimulation or Reuptake Inhibition	Clinical Consequence of Receptor Blockade	Common Uses of Medications in Class
Acetylcholine	Salivation, lacrimation, urination, diarrhea	Dry mouth, blurred vision, dry eyes, constipation	Xerostomia, memory, medication-induced or Parkinson's related tremors, cognition and global functioning in dementia
Norepinephrine	Tachycardia, increased blood pressure, blood vessel constriction	Bradycardia, decreased blood pressure, blood vessel dilation	Hypertension, depression
Epinephrine	Tachycardia, increased blood pressure, blood vessel constriction	Bradycardia, decreased blood pressure, blood vessel dilation	Asthma
Dopamine	Movement, euphoria, concentration	Abnormal movements, rigidity, tremors, postural imbalance, inattention	Motor symptoms of Parkinson's disease, schizophrenia, ADHD
Serotonin	Anxiety Insomnia Sexual dysfunction	Depression	Depression, anxiety, migraines, nausea
Histamine	Sneezing Wheezing Itching	Resolution of sneezing, wheezing, and itching	Allergies, GERD
Glutamate	Seizures	Sedation	Alzheimer's disease
Gamma Amino Butyric Acid	Sedation	Antiseizure, and anxiolytic affects	Seizures, anxiety

Sources: Adapted from Brenner & Stevens, 2006; Tiwari, Dwivedi, Singh, Mishra, & Changy, 2017; Li & Xu, 2008; Marieb, 2001; Berger, Gray, & Roth, 2009; Nieto-Alamilla, Marquez-Gomez, Garcia-Galvez, Morales-Figueroa, & Arias-Montano, 2016; Swanson, 2014; Meldrum, 2000; Monoghan, Bridges, & Cotman, 1989; Richelson & Souder, 2000.

Pharmacological Mechanisms of Medication-Induced Dysphagia

Swallowing is a complex process that involves both voluntary and reflexive motor activity, and there are multiple pharmacological mechanisms that impact these processes. The three primary pharmacological mechanisms that can lead to a dysphagia include: (1) inhibition or excitation of smooth muscle function during the oropharyngeal phase, (2) medication-induced esophageal injury, or (3) decrease of lower esophageal sphincter pressure. Dysphagia can also result when medications cause xerostomia (dry mouth) and/or dehydration (Al-Shehri, 2001; Balzer, 2000; Spieker, 2000). Additional mechanisms associated with dysphagia include muscle wasting, which is noted with high-dose steroids, and depressed immune function, which can be seen with the use of chemotherapeutic and other immunosuppressant agents (Balzer, 2000). When swallowing is impacted, individuals are subject to choking, aspiration pneumonia, malnutrition, dehydration, and/or weight loss.

Inhibition or Excitation of Smooth Muscle Function

Swallowing requires the inhibition and excitation of oropharyngeal muscles. These muscle sequences can be altered by various neurotransmitter mechanisms, as described below.

Acetylcholine/Cholinergic Mechanisms. Medications with cholinergic activity can excite smooth muscle function through their stimulating activity on acetylcholine receptors. Acetylcholine is a major neurotransmitter that is released by motor neurons, which modulate smooth muscle function. When acetylcholine is released, activation of muscles occurs, in addition to bodily processes such as salivation, urination, lacrimation, and digestion. Acetylcholine also influences cognitive processes, such as learning and memory. Medications that block the activity of acetylcholine are referred to as anticholinergic medications, and can cause the opposite of the previously mentioned effects to occur, such as blurred vision, constipation, sedation, confusion, and so forth. Anticholinergic medications are often used in Parkinson's disease (i.e., trihexyphenidyl, benztropine), asthma (i.e., ipratropium, tiotropium), and urinary incontinence (i.e., oxybutynin, tolteridine). Anticholinergic medications can affect deglutition by affecting

the cricopharyngeal muscles during the esophageal phase (Collamati et al., 2016; Leon, 2011; Spieker, 2000). In addition to affecting swallowing, anticholinergic medications can also cause xerostomia or dry mouth, which can impair the ability to move food around in the mouth (Bostock, Soiza, & Mangoni, 2010; Cochburn, Pradham, Taing, Kisley, & Ford, 2017; Marcum et al., 2016; Ruxton, Wood, & Mangoni, 2015). Medications that block histamine receptors, such as diphenhydramine or chlorpheniramine, can have similar effects on the oral, pharyngeal, or esophageal phases of swallowing (Tan, Lexomboon, Sandborgh-Englund, Haasum, & Johnell, 2018).

Antidopaminergic Mechanisms. Antipsychotic medications, otherwise known as neuroleptics, typically have antidopaminergic properties. These medications can negatively affect smooth muscle movement (Rudolph, 2017). Because of the high density of D2 receptors on smooth muscle, antipsychotics can cause extrapyramidal motor disturbances as a result of their D2 receptor-blocking pharmacology (Dayalu & Chou, 2008). The extrapyramidal effects can result in generalized motor disturbance, as well as dysphagia, impairing the function of striated musculature of the oropharynx and esophagus during the swallowing process (Al-Shehri, 2001).

There are two types of dysphagia caused by antipsychotics: bradykinetic dysphagia and dyskinetic dysphagia. Bradykinetic dysphagia is associated with other extrapyramidal symptoms, such as bradykinesia and motor restlessness, and resembles the dysphagia seen in patients with Parkinson's disease. Dyskinetic dysphagia is typically associated with tardive dyskinesia. Thus, swallowing problems with dyskinetic dysphagia are the result of involuntary movements of the tongue, lip, and jaw (Dziewas et al., 2007).

The first-generation or typical antipsychotics (i.e., haloperidol, fluphenazine, thorazine) are more likely to cause dysphagia because of their affinity for blocking the dopamine receptors, compared to the second-generation or atypical agents (i.e., clozapine, olanzapine, quetiapine, and risperidone). The first-generation antipsychotics block D2 receptors, adrenergic receptors, and anticholinergic receptors at varying levels to achieve their antipsychotic effects. The resulting extrapyramidal side effects (EPS) include tremors, rigidity, postural imbalance, and gynecomastia. Conversely, the second-generation antipsychotics primarily block D1 and D3 receptors, as well as 5HT2 receptors, to improve the psychosis and address other symptoms of schizophrenia, such as flat affect, apathy, and amotivation (Khanna et al., 2014; Komassa et al., 2009; Richelson & Souder, 2000; Seeman, 2002; Strange, 2001). Consequently, there is less risk for side effects, such as EPS, tardive dyskinesia, QT prolongation (the onset of ventricular contraction and relaxation in the heart), or gynecomastia with the second generation agents, but they are unfortunately associated with a higher risk of metabolic syndrome, serotonin syndrome, and sudden cardiac death.

Although dysphagia can more likely occur with the first generation antipsychotics, such as haloperidol and trifluoperazine, there are increasing case reports of dysphagia occurring from the newer agents as well (Dziewas et al., 2007). For example, a 54-year-old male reportedly experienced dysphagia from aripiprazole (Lin, Lee, Liao, Chiu, & Hsu, 2012). There are also case reports of EPS-related dysphagia involving other second-generation agents, such as clozapine, and risperidone (Dziewas et al., 2007; Lin et al., 2012). For both medication classes, the dysphagia occurred between 4 days and 5 weeks of initial dosing of the antipsychotic. In all cases, cessation of therapy with substitution of a less potent antipsychotic, dose reduction, and/or feeding strategies resolved the dysphagia. Unfortunately, there are limited ways to reverse dyskinetic dysphagia or tardive dyskinesia, but

removing the offending agent or finding a less offensive agent, coupled with feeding strategies, may provide some benefit (Dziewas et al., 2007). The second-generation agents may have less risk for causing dyskinetic dysphagia (Correll, Leucht, & Kane, 2004).

Gamma-Aminobutyric Acid (GABA) Mechanisms. GABA and glutamate are the primary neurotransmitters that signal the neurons for electronic transmission with glutamate giving the "go" signal, and GABA giving the "stop" signal. Medications that stimulate GABA receptors such as lorazepam or alprazolam can impair swallowing through their inhibitory effects on esophageal smooth muscles, similar to the effects on parts of the larynx or inferior portion of the cricopharyngeal muscle. These medications can also affect level of arousal or, in certain cases, directly affect the brainstem swallowing function (Buchholz, 1995). Buchholz and colleagues reported two cases of dose-dependent pharyngeal paresis during treatment with alprazolam that resolved with cessation of treatment (Buchholz, Jones, & Neumann, 1994).

Adrenergic Mechanisms. It is less common for medications with adrenergic properties (working on adrenaline or noradrenaline), such as albuterol, to cause swallowing difficulty. Instead, these medications typically improve swallowing by mimicking norepinephrine and epinephrine, which can increase the constriction of the vasculature innervating smooth muscle function. However, there have been reports of cricopharyngeal dysfunction in patients with chronic obstructive pulmonary disease, a disorder for which adrenergic agents like albuterol are often used.

Medication-Induced Esophageal Injury

The second pharmacological mechanism that can lead to dysphagia is esophageal injury.

Medications can cause direct injury to the esophagus due to physiochemical properties that require individuals to adhere to particular administrative methods to avoid injury. For example, the bisphosphonates are orally administered medications used for the treatment of osteoporosis that need to be taken with a full glass of water to facilitate passage of the medication through the esophagus. Failure to do so can cause erosions, ulcerations, and inflammation of the esophagus (O'Neal & Remington, 2003). Patients are instructed to remain upright for at least 30 to 60 minutes after the administration of the bisphosphonate to further ensure that the medication does not get attached to the mucosa (Zografos, Georgiadon, Thomas, Kaltsas, & Digalakis, 2009). The bisphosphonates have also been associated with causing osteonecrosis of the jaw, which can also contribute to the development of dysphagia (Habib, 2017). Other medications that can cause direct injury to the esophagus include aspirin or acetyl-salicylic acid. Aspirin causes direct injury to the esophagus by inhibiting cyclooxygenase (COX), which is an enzyme that produces prostaglandins that cause swelling, inflammation, fever, and pain. The inhibition of COX prevents platelet aggregation by decreasing the production of thromboxane, which is a prostaglandin that protects the stomach and other mucosal areas from damage. The use of enteric-coated aspirin products allows intestinal absorption of aspirin that minimizes damage to the gastrointestinal track. The nonsteroidal medications (i.e., ibuprofen, indomethacin, and naproxen) can also similarly damage the gastric mucosa through their platelet-inhibiting effects (Speiker, 2000; Sugawa, Takekuma, Lucas, & Amamoto, 1997). This effect provides relief from rheumatoid arthritis, headaches, and in the case of aspirin, prevents strokes and heart attacks, but increases the risk of gastric mucosal and esophageal bleeding from direct con-

tact with these products (Vane, 1997, 2003). Some antibiotics (i.e., doxycycline, tetracycline, trimethoprim-sulfamethoxazole) must also be administered with a full glass of water to facilitate passage through the esophagus, but can also chelate or bind to vitamins like iron when coadministered, rendering them inactive (Speiker, 2000).

Decrease of Lower Esophageal Sphincter Pressure

The third pharmacological mechanism that can lead to dysphagia is lowering of esophageal sphincter pressure. The lower esophageal sphincter is responsible for allowing the passage of food from the esophagus to the stomach. The sphincter relaxes to allow the passage of food and it closes after food passes through to prevent the regurgitation of the stomach's contents. This closure prevents irritation to the esophagus that could be caused by the mixture of gastric acids, bile, and pepsin. Consequently, medications that lower esophageal sphincter pressure can increase the likelihood of reflux of undigested food. Lower esophageal sphincter pressure is regulated through cholinergic, noradrenergic, or other mechanisms involving nitric oxide, substance P, and vasoactive intestinal peptide (Cheatam & Wong, 2011; Spechler & Castell, 2001).

In sum, there are numerous medications that can lead to a dysphagia because of alterations of smooth muscle function, esophageal injury, or esophageal sphincter pressure changes, in addition to issues such as xerostomia. Collectively, more than 400 medications can cause dysphagia by any of these mechanisms (Brenner & Stevens, 2006; Sonies 1997); clinicians should be familiar with these medications, and educate patients about these risks. Table 4–3 provides examples of medications that can cause these swallowing difficulties.

Table 4–3. Mechanisms of Medications that Can Cause Swallowing Disorders

Medications That Can Cause Esophageal Injury	Medications That Can Cause Dysphagia	Medications That Lower Esophageal Sphincter Pressure	Medications That Can Cause Xerostomia
Bisphosphonates	Antipsychotics	Cholecystokinin	Antihistamines
• Alendronate	Anxiolytics	Secretin	• Diphenhydramine
Antibiotics	Sedatives	Progesterone	Anticholinergics
Ascorbic acid	Antihistamines	Glucagon	• Atropine, Scopolamine
Aspirin	Anticholinergics	Neurotensin	Antiemetics
Doxycycline	• Incontinence Medications	Vasoactive Intestinal Polypeptide	Antipsychotics
Ferrous sulfate			• Mellaril, Thorazine
Ibuprofen	Diuretics	Dopamine	
Indomethacin	Mucosal Anesthetics	Beta blockers/agonists	Antihypertensives
Phenylbutazone	Oncolytics	Calcitonin Gene Related Polypeptide	• Clonidine, Reserpine
Prednisone	• Vincristine		Bronchodilators
Potassium chloride		Atropine	Opiates
Quinidine		Scopolamine	Diuretics
Theophylline		Theophylline	Antiarrhythmics
Nonsteroidal products		Morphine	Antispasmodics
		Nitrates	ACE Inhibitors
		Calcium antagonists	

CASE: ORAL DYSPHAGIA WITH HEAD AND NECK CANCER

A 56-year-old male presents to a speech-language pathology clinic with a medical history significant for T2N1M0 lingual cancer (Figure 4–1) treated with surgical resection (partial glossectomy), chemotherapy (Erbitux®), and radiation (RT) approximately one year ago. Prior to treatment for his cancer, the patient received a PEG tube to facilitate maintaining adequate hydration and nutrition given the anticipated odynophagia (painful swallowing) he would experience postoperatively and postchemo-radiation. The patient reported immediate changes to swallowing function following cancer intervention; however, the PEG tube was removed and he was able to feed himself orally with diet modifications, (pureed solids), increased meals times and reports of diminished taste.

Upon presentation to the speech-language pathologist, the patient reported continued worsening of swallowing function in the year since he received the initial cancer treatments, and additionally

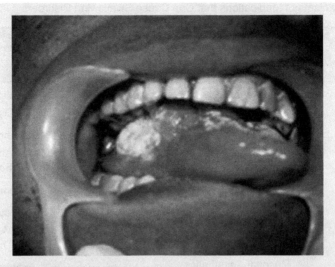

Figure 4–1. Patient with lingual cancer. *Source:* Image courtesy of USF Health.

acknowledged that he was unintentionally losing weight. The cranial nerve evaluation revealed markedly reduced range of motion of the lingual musculature, xerostomia, and mucositis; however, all other articulatory structures were within functional limits (WFL). A modified barium swallowing evaluation revealed a moderate-severe oral dysphagia characterized by difficulty with bolus formation, food pocketing in the cheeks, inadequate mastication, oral residue, difficulty with swallowing initiation, and slow oral transit time. The pharyngeal phase was functional for protection of the lower airways with no evidence of penetration, aspiration or significant vallecular or pyriform sinus residue.

Following the evaluation, the SLP educated the patient on some of the side effects of glossectomy, chemotherapy, as well as the often latent side effects of radiation, which likely explains his oral dysphagia, reduced lingual ROM, xerostomia, diminished taste, and mucositis. The clinician recommended that he participate in swallowing therapy to improve range of motion and

coordination of the lingual musculature during mastication and swallowing. Additionally, the patient was provided with recommendations for his xerostomia and mucositis, including use of Biotine® gum, increased water consumption, and the need to consult with his primary care physician regarding prescriptions for anti-inflammatory rinses, and so forth.

Discussion

Oral dysphagia has been found to impact more than 60% of patients treated with partial glossectomy in conjunction with chemoradiation intervention (D'Souza et al., 2007; Ihiara et al., 2018). This development of oral dysfunction results because of the critical role of the tongue for manipulation of solid food during mastication, safe bolus transport, and proper pressure generation to facilitate safe bolus transport through the pharynx. Chemotherapy and immunotherapy interventions are known to induce mucositis (painful tissue swelling and ulceration), dysgeusia (diminished taste), and copious secretions. Side effects of radiation therapy can also contribute to oral dysphagia. This treatment utilizes high-energy x-rays to kill cancer cells, which in turn reduces the size of a tumor. Some of the side effects of radiation affecting the mucosa and muscle tissue include xerostomia (chronic dry mouth), candidiasis (fungal infection) mucositis, fibrosis (stiffness/reduced ROM), and sensory changes to taste and smell.

Cetuximab (Erbitrux®) is an inhibitor of the epidermal growth factor, which is expressed in head and neck, colon, and rectum cancers. It is commonly prescribed with radiation therapy initially, used alone for locally or regionally advanced squamous, and various head and neck cancers (Erbitux Product Info, 2018). Dysphagia has been reported to have improved in patients with combination radiation and Cetumixab treatment (Liu & Wu, 2010; Tian, Zhou, Zeng, et al., 2015).

Pharmacological Management of Dysphagia

In some cases, medications like Botox or Botulinum toxin can prove beneficial in patients with dysphagia (Ahsan, Meleca, & Dworkin, 2000). Botox is an exotoxin that is produced in two types by the organism *Clostridium botulinum*. It was originally used in 1980 for strabismus, but then became a popular option to reduce wrinkles nearly a decade later. It was approved in 2002 as an alternative to cosmetic surgery, but has been used for numerous noncosmetic medical and surgical conditions, including dysphagia (Ahsan, et al., 2000; Graham et al., 2000; Heinen et al., 2010; Nayyar, Pravin, Nayyar, & Singh, 2014; Persaud et al., 2013; Zaninotto et al., 2004). Botulinum toxin A is used medicinally for blepharospasm, cervical dystonias, spasmodic dysphonias, migraines, and cosmetically to remove wrinkles. Botulinum toxin B is used for cervical dystonia.

Various health-related organizations have characterized the methodological quality of the studies of Botox for therapeutic purposes. Levels of study quality ranged from I to VII, with Level I suggesting the highest level of scientific rigor, such as randomized controlled trials, Level III comprised of cohort or case control studies, and Level IV including a case series (Ackley, Swan, Ladwig, & Tucker, 2008; Burns, Rohrich, & Chung, 2011; Sacket, 1989). According to the literature, there is Level I evidence for Botox for spasmodic dysphonia, essential voice tremor, and masticatory myalgia. There is Level II evidence for the effectiveness of Botox for vocal tics, dysphagia, and postlaryngectomy esophageal speech. Finally, there is Level IV evidence for stuttering, "first bite syndrome," oromandibular dystonia, and palatal/stapedial myoclonus (Persaud et al., 2013). For the studies of dysphagia, EMG-guided Botox injected into the cricopharyngeus muscle was found to be effective in several prospective and retrospective studies, but additional research is warranted.

Botox is typically injected into the cricopharyngeus muscle, upper esophageal sphincter, or other cervical muscles to reduce the spasms and hypertonicity associated with target muscle dysfunction. The therapeutic effects of Botox have been noted as early as 3 days after injection, and may last an average of 3 to 4 months, due to peripheral neuronal sprouting (Ahsan et al., 2000). Interestingly, Botox can also cause dysphagia in up to 33% of patients; it is thought that the dysphagia occurs because of the neuromuscular blockade, dosing, and/or site of injection (Comella,

Tanner, DeFoor-Hill, & Smith, 1992; Holzer & Ludlow, 1996; O'Neil & Remington, 2003). Botox acts locally at the neuromuscular junction by binding to cholinergic receptors and inhibiting the release of acetylcholine, resulting in paralysis of the injected muscle (Ahsan et al., 2000). Paralysis and total loss

of miniature end-plate potentials are evident after Botox injections. The following case demonstrates the importance of diagnostic considerations and the dosing of Botox appropriately.

Other medications that can be used to treat swallowing disorders include dopami-

---

CASE: PHARYNGEAL DYSPHAGIA FROM BOTOX INJECTION

A 65-year-old female presented emergently to an outpatient multidisciplinary neurology clinic for insidious decline of swallowing function following an injection of Botox the day before for the management of a voice disorder. The patient reported that she received a diagnosis of adductor spasmodic dysphonia one week prior from a community ENT, and subsequently decided to receive an injection of Botox into the intrinsic laryngeal thyroarytenoid muscles for treatment of the involuntary muscular contraction. However, immediately following her injection, the patient noticed constant coughing/choking on her saliva and any solids/liquids that she attempted to consume. Additionally, her voice became markedly breathy, and phonation became difficult. The patient denied using any additional pharmacological intervention that may have contributed to the onset of her voice disorder or swallowing dysfunction.

The patient was first evaluated by the SLP using a standard cranial nerve evaluation (all articulatory structures were within functional limits (WFL) for force, direction, range of motion (ROM), and speed in the oral and facial musculature), perceptual motor speech/voice evaluation, and various acoustic measures. Following these evaluative procedures, the patient received a transnasal flexible laryngoscopic evaluation which revealed immobility of her vocal folds during phonation and during attempted swallows of saliva, thin liquids, and pudding. In fact, the patient aspirated all attempted saliva and bolus swallows, which were immediately followed by aggressive reflex coughs. These results suggested a profound pharyngeal dysphagia in the absence of oral or esophageal stage deficits. The pharyngeal stage of swallowing is largely considered reflexive and under voluntary control. Safe transit of a bolus into the esophagus requires coordinated valving of the laryngeal mechanism and upper esophageal sphincter. As such, the intrinsic laryngeal muscles must adduct tightly in conjunction with laryngeal vestibule closure, epiglottic inversion, and pharyngeal peristalsis while the cricopharyngeal muscle relaxes to allow passage of bolus material into the esophagus. Too much Botox or improper placement of the Botox was likely the cause of such marked paralysis of the vocal folds.

Given the severity of the patient's pharyngeal dysphagia and the relatively long-term effects of Botox for muscular paralysis, the patient was recommended to receive immediate placement of a PEG tube for maintenance of hydration and nutrition. She was educated that the side effects of the Botox would persist for approximately

3 to 4 months, at which time her voice and swallowing function would likely return to baseline. The patient returned to the clinic when the Botox effects wore off and it was determined that she had received an improper diagnosis of spasmodic dyspho- nia and, in fact, had an essential tremor of the larynx. A repeat laryngoscopic evalua- tion revealed resolution of her pharyngeal dysphagia, and the PEG tube was removed. She initiated behavioral voice therapy for management of her laryngeal tremor.

nergic stimulating agents, such as ropin- orole, pramipexole, or levodopa/carbidopa in patients with Parkinson's disease (Tolosa, Martí, Valldeoriola, & Molinuevo, 1998). These agents facilitate the restoration of smooth muscle function through the release of dopamine in the *substantia nigra* by stimulat- ing various dopamine receptors. Because these receptors are predominantly centrally located, the use of these agents as primary treatment for dysphagia is not commonplace, but they have proven to be beneficial in treating trem- ors, rigidity, and postural imbalance associated with Parkinson's disease (Fox et al., 2018). Patients with Parkinson's disease can have difficulty swallowing foods and medications, purportedly because of the rigidity and brady- kinesia associated with the disease. Thus, the dopamine agonists may be beneficial in these patients, but additional research is warranted.

Strategies for Clinicians to Address Medication-Induced Swallowing Difficulty

Clinicians can utilize various strategies to min- imize the effects of medications that cause dys- phagia. Changing solid formulations to liquid preparations, or using oral dispersible formula- tions, is one mechanism that can be consid-ered when medications cause swallowing difficulty (Kelly, D'Cruz, & Wright, 2010; Kirke-vold & Engedal, 2010). When this strategy is uti- lized, clinicians should pay close attention to dosing equivalences between the formula- tions. Thickening liquid medications can help prevent aspiration. Another strategy is to em- ploy alternate or nonoral routes of adminis- tration like the intranasal, transdermal, paren- teral, enteral, or buccal route. When adminis- tering medications by the parenteral or enteral route, a functional gastrointestinal tract is required, timely flushing of tubes is needed, and special attention is required to minimize medication interactions. When using oral dis- persible products, clinicians should make sure that patients do not have allergies to phenyl- alanine and other ingredients that facilitate the dispensability of the medication.

Patients with dysphagia, and very often, individuals who are elderly, have difficulty administering solid dosage forms effectively, so alternate formulations may need to be con- sidered (Schiele, Quinzler, Klimm, Pruszy- dlo, & Haefeli, 2013). When medications are not available in nonoral solid dosage forms, crushing or otherwise altering non-extended- release medications may also be an option to minimize swallowing difficulty. Manipula- tions of tablet and capsules include splitting, tablet crushing, or dispersion or dissolution of the tablet/capsule content in cold liquids or semisolid foods, such as pudding (Haw & Stubbs, 2010). Solid oral dosage formula- tions may be scored to facilitate their splitting. Manipulation of the original dosage form can sometimes cause adverse effects and negatively impact therapeutic outcomes (Kelly, Wright, & Wood, 2011). Table 4–4 highlights some medication formulations that should not be crushed or altered (Cornish, 2005).

Table 4–4. Medication Formulations That Should Not Be Crushed or Altered

Type of Formulation	Common Terms and Abbreviations	Purpose of the Formulation
Enteric-Coated	Delayed-release Enteric Coated	Designed to pass through the stomach intact and to be delivered into the intestine because: • The medication is unstable in gastric acid • The medication irritates the stomach • The onset of action is intended to be delayed
Extended-Release	CD: Controlled Delivery CR: Controlled Release LA: Long Acting PA: Prolonged Action SR: Slow Release SR: Sustained Release XL: Extended Release XR: Extended Release	Designed for the dosage form to release the medication over an extended period of time. Formulations include: • Multiple-layered tablets that release the medication as each layer is dissolved • Mixed release granules • Inert matrices to allow slow release of the medication

Formulations for Patients With Dysphagia

There are various types of drug formulations, such as solutions, suspensions, orally dissolving tablets (ODTs), and chewable tablets. Each formulation is unique and requires a careful preparation processes. A formulation preference study carried out by Wright and colleagues showed that patients with dysphagia preferred liquid medicines and tablets with coated, torpedo shapes (Wright, Jarrman, Connolly, & Dissmann, 2009). If a patient has dysphagia for liquids, then the viscosity of the liquid preparations should be taken into account, and tablets would be a better option.

Clinicians should inquire about any difficulty in swallowing medications as a part of all clinical evaluations. Prescribers should take into consideration the degree of swallowing impairment to determine the appropriate formulation of the medication, and the pharmacists can further assess the suitability of particular formulations for the individual patients. Patients and caregivers should also provide input when swallowing difficulties arise. Efforts must also be made to discern the degree of impact on feeding, and other quality of life issues. Ensuring that patients get adequate hydration, minimizing the number of medications being taken, and incorporating mucolytics, when necessary (i.e., agents that dissolves thick mucus), are additional strategies that can be considered to minimize dysphagia (Kelly & Wright, 2009; Kirkevold & Engedal, 2010; Kyle, 2011; O'Neal & Remington, 2003). The algorithm in Figure 4–2 can be used by clinicians to determine strategies to prevent or resolve medication-related swallowing disorders.

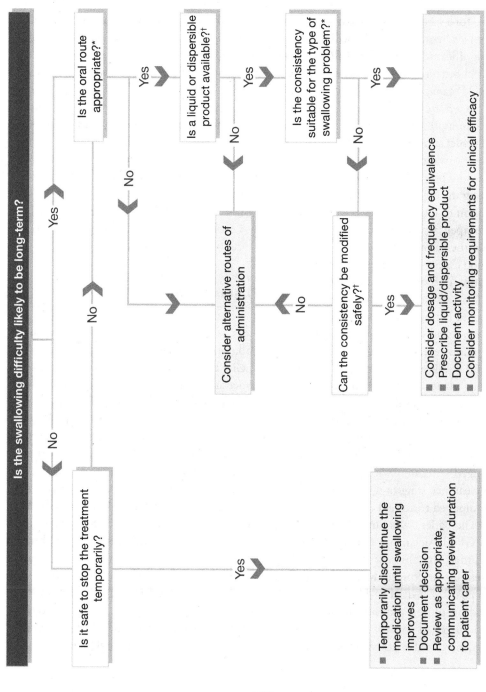

Figure 4–2. Algorithm for the medication management of adults with swallowing difficulties. *Source:* Adapted from Wright, D., Begent, D., Crawford, H., Foundling-Miah, M., Griffith, R., & Merriman, H., 2018, Medication management of adults with swallowing difficulties. In N. Hayeem (Ed.). *Guidelines—summarising clinical guidelines for primary care* (68th ed., pp. 65–68). Chesham, UK: MGP Ltd. Available at http://www.guidelines.co.uk/dysphagia/swallowing-difficulties-medication-management-guideline/453844.article Reproduced with permission.

Seek advice from:
* Speech-language pathologist +/– occupational therapist, physical therapist, dietician (if involved in dysphagia management).
† Supplying pharmacist and/or Medicines Information Centre.

CASE: ESOPHAGEAL DYSPHAGIA

A 26-year-old male with a history of progressive swallowing difficulty, primarily with solid foods more than liquids, presented for a speech-language pathology outpatient evaluation. His past medical history was significant for asthma and allergies, elevated cholesterol and blood pressure, and GERD, managed with daily oral medication (omeprazole).

Upon presentation to the SLP, the patient's chief complaints included significant difficulty swallowing tough meats, breads, salads, and pills; intermittent coughing and choking during meal times; and a frequent sensation of food at the level of the throat. To compensate for these swallowing difficulties the patient reported that he chewed his food excessively in hopes of avoiding the sensation of food in the pharynx.

The patient was evaluated using a modified barium swallowing evaluation in the lateral and anterior viewing planes. The evaluation revealed normal oral and pharyngeal swallowing function in the lateral viewing planes, with no evidence of airway compromise or residue.

A brief scan of the esophagus in the anterior view revealed residue in the esophagus, and eosinophilic esophagitis (EoE), or a "ringed stricture," with delayed esophageal clearance (Figure 4–3). EoE is caused by prolonged treatment of GERD.

The patient was immediately referred to a GI physician for management who concluded that his condition was likely caused by prolonged history of asthma and possibly GERD. The patient was placed on proton pump inhibitor therapy and an ingested corticosteroid. After a few weeks, he noted marked improvement of his symptoms. The patient returned to the SLP clinic for dysphagia counseling and education to reduce and prevent the signs and symptoms of his esophageal dysphagia moving forward. In addition to medication management for EoE, the patient received the following behavioral recommendations:

- Remain in an upright position during and after meals for at least 10 to 45 minutes.
- Alternate solids and liquids during meals.
- Drink 2 to 3 ounces of liquid per pill to be swallowed.
- Oval, small, and coated pills are better.
- Crush medications as needed or mix in a viscous material when able.

Discussion

EoE is a condition caused by chronic inflammation and thickening of the epithelial cells in the esophagus that leads to mucosal and smooth muscle hypertrophy, cellular proliferation, loss of elasticity, stenosis, and fragility of the tissue. Dysphagia is a prominent symptom in adolescents, but children typically present with other manifestations, such as food allergies, asthma, eczema, chronic rhinitis, and environmental allergies. GERD and heartburn are commonly seen as well. EoE typically presents during childhood, or the third or fourth decade of life, but can occur at any age. Dysphagia may be accompanied by chest pain, food impaction, and upper abdominal pain; however, solid-food dysphagia continues to be the most common presentation (Liacaouras et al., 2011).

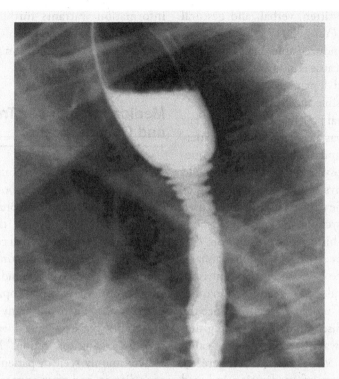

Figure 4–3. Eosinophilic esophagitis. This figure illustrates eosinophilic esophagitis (EoE) that was identified during a brief anterior view videofluoroscopic scan of the esophagus. *Source:* Image courtesy of USF Health.

The goals for treating EoE are to control the esophageal eosinophilia and inflammation. Treatment of EoE is typically managed with proton pump inhibitors for 8 to 12 weeks, topical or oral corticosteroids, and dietary therapy (Liacaouras et. al. 2011; Straumann & Katska, 2018).

EoE is also an opportunity for prescribers to pay attention to the formulations of medications being used in patients with this disease, and demonstrates the utility of crushing medications, and other medication administration techniques.

MEDICATION-INDUCED LANGUAGE, SPEECH, AND COGNITIVE DISORDERS

Medications can also cause or complicate cognitive-communication disorders. Several examples are provided below.

Aphasia

Aphasia is the inability to comprehend and formulate language as a consequence of damage to certain regions in the brain. It commonly occurs following strokes, but can also emerge after infections, head trauma, and/or tumors. Aphasia is a multimodality disorder and can affect written, verbal, and gestural communication (Yang, 2017). Like dysphagia, medication-induced aphasia has also been noted. The exact cause is unknown, but central neurotoxicity and dopamine-blocking activity are but two possible mechanisms that interact with individual patient characteristics. For example, there was a case report of the emergence of global aphasia from the use of quetiapine (an antipsychotic) in an 83-year-old female after 3 days of use (Chien, Huang & Hsieh, 2017). The patient had previously used a different antipsychotic medication (Risperidone) and had a history of hypertension, diabetes, and a prior stroke. The global aphasia persisted for three days, and a transient ischemic attack was ruled out, in addition to other medical causes. The aphasia resolved once the quetiapine was discontinued, suggesting that the quetiapine was the contributing cause (Chien, Huang, & Hsieh, 2017). There are other case reports of medication-induced aphasia related to the use of lamotrigine, vigabatrin, cisplatin, sulfasalazine, ifosfamide, and phenylpropanolamine, to name a few (Chien et al., 2017).

Stuttering

Medication-induced stuttering has also been reported in the literature. A total of 51 cases of medication-induced stuttering were reported in the French Pharmacovigilance Database between 1985 and 2014. There were seven cases involving antiepileptics, six involving antipsychotics, five cases involving antidepressants, two cases involving antihistamines and anticancer therapies, and one case involving a vaccine, antibiotic, immunosuppressive, or TNF-an antagonist. The onset of the stuttering ranged between one and three years, and improvement was noted in 32 of the cases with stopping or reducing the dose of the medication (Bene et al., 2014). However, this information warrants further investigation considering the range in onset of symptoms and response to medication elimination or dosage reduction.

Medication-Induced Tremors and Communication

Tremors are defined as involuntary, rhythmic, oscillatory movement of a body part such as hands, legs, neck, and jaw (Bhatia et al., 2017; Dayalou & Chou, 2008), thus potentially impacting written and verbal communication. Tremors are the most common movement disorder and a key extrapyramidal side effect of antipsychotics and other dopamine-blocking medications. There are many different types of tremors, but one general way to categorize them is "resting" or "action." Resting tremors are commonly seen in patients with Parkinson's disease, and often appear as a pill-rolling motion of the hand that disappears upon voluntary movement. Action tremors, in contrast, are tremors that occur with voluntary movement, for example while writing, drawing, typing, shaving, or brushing the teeth (Bhatia et al., 2017; Mailankody, Netravanthi, & Pal, 2017; NINDS Factsheet on Tremors). Vocal tremors can also occur, and can result in an unsteady voice. Both resting and action tremors can be caused or exacerbated by medications.

Risk factors for tremors include genetic mutations and age, which is the most important risk factor for development of a medication-induced tremor (Morgan & Sethi, 2005). This is attributed to the increased rate of medication-disease interactions (for example, the presence of renal failure or liver failure) with age. Polypharmacy, mood, and anxiety also play a role in the manifestation and severity of medication-induced tremors in the elderly. Table 4–5 outlines medications that can cause tremors.

Table 4–5. Medications That Cause Tremors

Drug Class	Specific Offenders
Antiarrhythmics	Amiodarone, mexiletine, procainamide
Antibiotics	Co-trimoxazole, amphotericin B
Antidepressants and mood stabilizers	Amitriptyline, lithium, SSRIs
Antiepileptics	Valproic acid
Bronchodilators	Salbutamol, salmeterol
Chemotherapeutics	Tamoxifen, cytarabine, ifosfamide, thalidomide
Gastrointestinal agents	Metoclopramide, cimetidine
Hormones	Thyroxine, calcitonin, medroxyprogesterone, epinephrine
Immunosuppressants	Tacrolimus, cyclosporine, interferon-alpha
Methylxanthines	Theophylline, caffeine
Antipsychotics	Haloperidol

Table 4–6 outlines additional questions to integrate into the evaluation process in the case of a suspected medication-induced tremor. Imaging, laboratory testing, and other measures should also be implemented as necessary to determine the cause and treatment plan.

Cognitive Deficits

Medications can affect cognitive processing by causing confusion, sedation, amnesia, and delirium. Almost 10% of commonly used drugs among cognitively normal adults have been associated with longitudinal changes in cognition (Obermann, Morris, & Roe, 2013). Anticholinergic medications, in particular, have been linked to impaired cognition in older adults, particularly in immediate memory recall and executive functions, as well as whole-brain and temporal lobe atrophy (Risacher et al., 2016). These findings highlight the importance of the cholinergic system in cognition and suggest that medications with anticholinergic properties may be detrimental to brain structure and function, in addition to cognition (Risacher et al., 2016).

Antihistamines, benzodiazepines, sedative hypnotics, analgesics, urinary agents, gastrointestinal agents, and some antipsychotics can also cause confusion and sedation. The benzodiazepines can cause retrograde amnesia in addition to sedation (Collamati et al., 2016; Ham, Agostini, & Allore, 2008; Ruxton et al., 2015; Sittironnarit et al., 2011). Examples of medications that have cognitive-impairing effects are listed in Table 4–7. There are nonprescription products used for sleep and allergies that contain antihistamines and analgesics, which can also cause sedation or confusion. Additionally, herbal products, such as chamomile, kava kava, valerian, and melatonin can cause sedation and confusion (Hussin, 2001; Sarris & McIntyre, 2017).

Table 4–6. Treatment Questions to Consider if Concern for Medication-Induced Tremor

Treatment Question	Rationale
Is the tremor bothersome to the patient in social or occupational functioning?	Most medication-induced tremors are mild and determining impact is prudent.
Is the medication essential for the patient? If so, are there possible alternative medication options?	Some medical disorders require treatment, despite the side effects, and selection of an alternative therapy with less likelihood to cause tremors should be considered. For example, discontinuing metoclopramide and replacing with erythromycin for gastroparesis.
Can the dose of the medication be lowered?	Dose reductions may not necessarily decrease the efficacy of the therapy, but may lessen the side effect of tremor. Careful monitoring for maintained efficacy is warranted.
Can a medication be added to mask the tremor due to the first medication?	Sometimes, if treatment with the medication of concern cannot be modified, addition of another medication (e.g., propranolol for a medication-induced resting tremor) may yield benefit.
Can occupational therapy and lifestyle adaptation improve the patient's quality of life?	If medication therapy modification or cessation is not successful, occupational therapy may be able to assist with introduction of weighted utensils or other adaptive equipment.

Source: Adapted from Morgen and Sethi, 2005.

Table 4–7. Examples of Prescription Medications That Can Cause Cognitive Impairment

Mechanism of Cognitive Impairment	Classes of Medications
Sedation	Antihistamines, anticholinergics, benzodiazepines, antipsychotics, nonbenzodiazepine sedative hypnotics, barbiturates, urinary incontinence agents, antidepressants, analgesics
Confusion	Antihistamine, urinary incontinence agents, antipsychotics, cardiovascular agents, analgesics
Amnesia	Benzodiazepines, gastrointestinal agents
Delirium	Anticholinergics, opioid analgesics, benzodiazepine and nonbenzodiazepine sedative hypnotics

Cognitive challenges are characteristic of many neurological and medical disorders; therefore, it can be difficult to determine whether a medication is responsible for a change to cognition. Understanding the timing of medication use can be helpful. For instance, sedation is especially notable at the initiation of a medication or following a dosage change (Johnson, 2013). However, medication use can also have a detrimental effect on cognition over time. For example, long-term stimulant prescription use was associated with worsening symptoms of hyperactivity, impulsivity, and learning problems in children aged 3 to 19 with perinatal HIV (Sirois et al., 2016). Because of the shared clinical presentation, clinicians will need to rule out disorders such as strokes, which can also cause confusion and memory impairment. SLPs should also be aware of the impact of other contributors to decreased cognition, such as compromised sleep, chronic stress, and dehydration. Overall, given the complexity of medication influence and interactions, SLPs will need a strong working relationship with the pharmacist and consulting physician.

In conclusion, medications can contribute to the emergence or exacerbation of swallowing and cognitive-communication disorders. Clinicians should be mindful of selecting appropriate formulations and instituting strategies to minimize this risk.

Key Resources

American Speech Language Hearing Association: http://www.asha.org

Dysphagia Research Society http://www.dysphagiaresearch.org

National Foundation of Swallowing Disorders: http://www.swallowing disorderfoundation.com

Medline Plus: http://Medlineplus.gov/swallowingdisorders.html

http://Swallowstudy.com/medication-induced-dysphagia-resources-safe-practices

http://Thickit.com

REFERENCES

Ackley, B., Swan, B., Ladwig, G., & Tucker S. (2008). *Evidence-based nursing care guidelines: Medical-surgical interventions.* St. Louis, MO: Mosby Elsevier.

Ahsan, S., Meleca, R., & Dworkin, J. (2000). Botulinum toxin injection of the cricopharyngeus muscle for the treatment of dysphagia. *Otolaryngology-Head and Neck Surgery, 122,* 691–695.

Alomar, M. (2014). Factors affecting the development of adverse drug reactions (Review article). *Saudi Pharmaceutical Journal, 22*(2), 83–94.

Al-Shehri, A. (2003). Dysphagia as a medication side effect. *Internet Journal of Otorhinolaryngology, 1*(2), 1–9.

Balzer, K. (2000). Medication-induced dysphagia. *International Journal of MS Care, 2*(1), 40–50.

Bene, J., Auffret, M., Fedrizzi, F., Valnet-Rabier, M. B., Caron, J., Gautier, S. & the French Association of Regional Pharmacovigilance Centres. (2014). *Medication-induced stuttering: A review of the French pharmacovigilance database.* Centre Hospitalier Regional Universitaire de Lille ISOP 2014. P088.

Benet, L. Z., & Hoener, B. A. (2002). Changes in plasma protein binding have little clinical relevance. *Clinical Pharmacology and Therapeutics, 71,* 115–221.

Berger, M., Gray, J, & Roth, B. (2009). The expanded biology of serotonin. *Annual Review of Medicine, 60,* 355–366.

Bhatia, K., Bain, P., Bajaj, N., Elble, R. J., Hallett, M., Louis, E. D., . . . Deuschl, G. (2017). Consensus statement on the classification of tremors, from the task force on tremor of the IPMDS. *Movement Disorders, 33*(1), 75–87.

Billioti de Gage, S., Bégaud, B., Bazin, F., Verdoux, H., Dartigues, J. F., Perex, K., . . . Pariente, A. (2012). Benzodiazepine use and risk of dementia: Prospective population based study. *British Medical Journal, 345–357,* e6231.

Bostock, C., Soiza, R., & Mangoni, A. A. (2010). Association between prescribing of antimuscarinic medications and antimuscarinic adverse effects in older people. *Expert Review of Clinical Pharmacology, 3*(4), 441–452.

Brenner, G., & Stevens, C. (2006). *Pharmacology* (2nd ed.). Philadelphia, PA: W.B. Saunders.

Buchholz, D. (1995). Dysphagia oropharyngeal dysphagia due to iatrogenic neurological dysfunction. *Dysphagia, 10*(4), 248–254.

Buchholz, D., Jones, B., & Neumann, W. (1994). *Two cases of benzodiazepine-induced pharyngeal dysphagia.* Presented at the Dysphagia Research Society Conference, McLean, Virginia.

Burns, P., Rohrich, R., & Chung, K. (2011). The levels of evidence and their role in evidence-based medicine. *Plastic and Reconstructive Surgery, 128*(1), 305–310.

Cheatham, J., & Wong, R. (2011). Current approach to the treatment of achalasia. *Current Gastroenterology Reports, 13*(3), 219–225.

Chien, C., Huang, P., & Hsieh, S. (2017). Reversible global aphasia as a side effect of quetiapine: A case report and literature review. *Neuropsychiatric Disease and Treatment, 13*, 2257–2260.

Cochburn, N., Pradham, A., Taing, M., Kisely, S., & Ford, P. J. (2017). Oral health impacts of medications used to treat mental illness. *Journal of Affective Disorders, 223*, 184–193.

Collamati, A., Martone, A., Poscia, A., Brandi, V., Celi, M., Marzetti, E., . . . Landi, F. (2016). Anticholinergic medications and negative outcomes in the older population: From biological plausibility to clinical evidence. *Aging Clinical and Experimental Research, 28*(1), 25–35.

Comella, C., Tanner, C., DeFoor-Hill, L., & Smith, C. (1992). Dysphagia after botulinum toxin injections for spasmodic torticollis: Clinical and radiologic findings. *Neurology, 42*, 1307–1310.

Cornish, P. (2005). "Avoid the crush": Hazards of medication administration in patients with dysphagia or a feeding tube. *Canadian Medical Association Journal, 172*(7), 871–872.

Correll, C., Leucht, S., & Kane, J. (2004). Lower risk for tardive dyskinesia associated with second-generation antipsychotics: A systemic review of 1-year studies. *American Journal of Psychiatry, 161*, 414.

Dayalou, P., & Chou, K. (2008). Antipsychotic-induced extrapyramidal symptoms and their management. *Expert Opinion on Pharmacotherapy, 9*(9), 1451–1462.

D'Souza, G., Kreimer, A., Viscidi, R., Pawliti, M., Fahkry, C., Koch, W., . . . Gillison M. (2007). Case-control study of human papillomavirus and oropharyngeal cancer. *New England Journal of Medicine, 356*, 1944–1956.

Dziewas, R., Warnecke, T., Schnabel, M., Ritter, M., Nabavi, D., Schilling, M, . . . Reker, T. (2007). Neuroleptic-induced dysphagia: Case report and literature review. *Dysphagia, 22*, 63–67.

Erbitux Product Info Labeling. ImClone LLC. (2018, June).

Fox, S., Katzenschlager, R., Lim, S., Barton, B., de Bie, R., Seppi, K., . . . Sampaio, C. (2018). International Parkinson and Movement Disorder Society evidence-based medicine review: Update on treatments for the motor symptoms of Parkinson's disease. *Movement Disorders. 33*(8), 1248–1266.

Fusco, S., Cariati, D., Schepisi, R., Ganzetti, R., Sestili, M., David, S., . . . Corica, F. (2016). Management of oral medication therapy in elderly patients with dysphagia. *Journal of Gerontology & Geriatrics, 64*, 9–20.

Graham, H., Aoki, K., Autti-Ramo, I., Boyd, R. N., Delgado, M. R., Gaebler-Spira, D. J., . . . Wissel J. (2000). Recommendations for the use of botulinum toxin type A in the management of cerebral palsy. *Gait Post, 11*(1), 67–79.

Habib, Z. (2017). Bisphosphonates in the treatment of osteoporosis: A review of skeletal safety concerns. *Expert Review of Endocrinology & Metabolism, 12*, 59–71.

Hajjar, E., Cafiero, A., & Hanlon, J. T. (2007). Polypharmacy in elderly patients. *American Journal of Geriatric Pharmacotherapy, 5*(4), 345–351.

Ham, L., Agostini, J., & Allore, H. (2008). Cumulative anticholinergic exposure is associated with poor memory and executive function in older men. *Journal of the American Geriatric Society, 56*(12), 2203–2210.

Hara, K., Tohara, H., Kobayashi, K., Yamaguchi, K., Yoshimi, K., Nakane, A., & Minakuchi, S. (2018). Age-related declines in the swallowing muscle strength of men and women aged 20–89 years: A cross-sectional study on tongue pressure and jaw-opening force in 980 subjects. *Archives of Gerontology and Geriatrics, 78*, 64–70.

Haw, C., & Stubbs, J. (2010). Administration of medicines in food and drink: A study of older inpatients with severe mental illness. *International Psychogeriatrics, 22*(3), 409–416.

Heinen, F., Desloovere, K., Schroeder, A., Berweck, S., Borggraefe, I., van Campenhaut A., . . . Molenaers G. (2010). The updated European consensus 2009 on the use of botulinum toxin for children with cerebral palsy. (2010). *European Journal of Peadiatric Neurology, 14*(1), 45–66.

Holzer, S., & Ludlo, C. (1996). The swallowing side effects of botulinum toxin type A injection in spasmodic dysphonia. *Laryngoscope, 106,* 86–92.

Hussin, J. (2001). Adverse effects of herbals and drug-herbal interactions. *Malaysian Journal of Pharmacy, 1*(2), 39–44.

Ihara, Y., Crary, M., Madhavan, A., Gregorio, D. C., Im, I., Ross, S. E., & Carnaby, G. D. (2018). Dysphagia and oral morbidities in chemoradiation-treated head and neck cancer patients. *Dysphagia, 33*(6), 739–748.

Jankovic, J., & Schwartz, K. (1991). Botulinum toxin treatment of tremors. *Neurology, 41*(8), 1185. https://doi.org/10.1212/WNL.41.8.1185

Johnson, P. R. (2013). The effects of medications on cognition in long-term care. *Seminars in Speech and Language, 34,* 18–28.

Kelly, J., & Wright, D. (2009). Administering medication to adult patients with dysphagia. *Nursing Standards, 23,* 62–68.

Kelly, J., D'Cruz, G., & Wright, D. (2009). A qualitative study of the problems surrounding medicine administration to patients with dysphagia. *Dysphagia, 24,* 49–56.

Kelly, J., D'Cruz, G., & Wright, D. (2010). Patients with dysphagia: Experiences of taking medication. *Journal of Advanced Nursing, 66,* 82–91.

Kelly, J., Wright, D., & Wood, J. (2011). Medicine administration errors in patients with dysphagia in secondary care: A multi-centre observational study. *Journal of Advanced Nursing, 67*(12), 2615–2627.

Khanna, P., Suo, T., Komassa, K., Ma, H., Rummel-Kluge, C., El-Sayeh, H. G., . . . Xia, J. (2014). Aripiprazole versus other atypical antipsychotics for schizophrenia. *Cochrane Database of Systematic Reviews, 2014*(1), CD006569.

Kirkevold, O., & Engedal, K. (2010). What is the matter with crushing pills and opening capsules? *International Journal of Nursing Practice, 16,* 81–85.

Komossa, K., Rummel-Kluge, C., Schmid, F., Hunger, H., Schwarz, S., El-Sayeh, H. G., . . . Leucht, S. (2009). Aripiprazole versus other atypical antipsychotics for schizophrenia. *Cochrane Database of Systematic Reviews, 2009*(4), CD006569.

Kouladjian, L., Gnjidic, D., Reeve, E., Chen, T. F., & Hilmer, S. N. (2016). Health care practitioners' perspectives on deprescribing anticholinergic and sedative medications in older adults. *Annals of Pharmacotherapy, 50*(8), 625–636.

Krishnakanth, M., Phutane, V. H., & Muralidharan, K. (2008). Clozapine-induced stuttering: A case series. *Primary Care Companion to the Journal of Clinical Psychiatry, 10,* 333–334.

Kumar, T., Kathpal, A., & Longshore C. (2013). Dose dependent stuttering with clozapine: A case report. *Asian Journal of Psychiatry, 6*(2), 178–179.

Kyle, G. (2011). Managing dysphagia in older people with dementia. *British Journal of Community Nursing, 16,* 6–10.

Lader, M. (2011). Benzodiazepines revisited—will we ever learn? *Addiction, 106*(12), 2086–2109.

Lalonde, R. (1985). Dopaminergic supersensitivity after long-term administration of phenytoin in rats. *Epilepsia, 26*(1), 81–84.

Landi, F., Dell'Aquila, G., Collamati, A., Martone, A. M., Zuliani, G., Gasperini, B, . . . Cherubini, A. (2014). Anticholinergic medication use and negative outcomes among the frail elderly population living in a nursing home. *Journal of the American Medical Directors Association, 15*(11), 825–829.

Leon, J. D. (2011). Paying attention to pharmacokinetic and pharmacodynamic mechanisms to progress in the area of anticholinergic use in geriatric patients. *Current Medication Metabolism, 12*(7), 635–646.

Liacaouras, C., Furuta, G., Hirano, I., Atkins, D., Attwood, S. E., Bonis, P. A., . . . Aceves, S. S. (2011). Eosinophillic esophagitis: Updated consensus recommendations for children and adults. *Journal of Allergy and Clinical Immunology, 128*(1), 3–20.

Li, K., & Xu, E. (2008). The role and the mechanism of γ-aminobutyric acid during central nervous system development. *Neuroscience Bulletin, 24*(3), 195–200.

Lin, T. W., Lee, B., Liao, Y. C., Chui, N. Y., & Hsu, W. Y. (2012). High dosage of aripiprazole-induced dysphagia. *International Journal of Eating Disorders, 45*(2), 305–306

Liu, H., & Wu, G. (2010). Clinical effect and life quality of radiotherapy combined with Erbitux in the treatment of advanced esophageal carcinoma.

Mailankody, P., Netravanthi, M., & Pal, P. (2017). Review of tremor in Parkinson's disease and atypical parkinsonian disorders. *Neurology India, 65,* 1083–1090.

Mangoni, A., & Jackson, S. (2003). Age-related changes in pharmacokinetics and pharmacodynamics: Basic principles and practical applications. *British Journal of Clinical Pharmacology, 57*(1), 6–14.

Marcum, Z. A., Wirtz, H. S., Pettinger, M., LaCroix A. Z., Carnahan, R., Cauley, J. A., . . . Gray, S. L. (2016). Anticholinergic medication use and falls in postmenopausal women: Findings from the women's health initiative cohort study. *BMC Geriatrics, 16*(1), 76.

Marieb, E. (2001). *Human anatomy & physiology.* San Francisco, CA: Benjamin Cummings.

Meldrum, B. (2000). Glutamate as a neurotransmitter in the brain: Review of physiology and pathology. *Journal of Nutrition, 130*(4S Suppl.), 1007S–1015S.

Molfenter, S. M., Brates, D., Herzberg, E., Noorani, M., & Lazarus, C. (2018). The swallowing profile of healthy aging adults: Comparing noninvasive swallow tests to videofluoroscopic measures of safety and efficiency. *Journal of Speech, Language, and Hearing Research, 61*(7), 1603–1612.

Monoghan, D., Bridges, J., & Cotman, C. (1989). The excitatory amino acid receptors: Their classes, pharmacology, and distinct properties in the function of the central nervous system. *Annual Review of Pharmacology Toxicology, 29,* 365–402.

Morgan, J., & Sethi, K. (2005). Medication-induced tremors. *Lancet Neurology, 4,* 866–876.

Nayyar, P, Pravin, K., Nayyar, P., & Singh, A. (2014). Botox: Broadening the horizon of dentistry. *Journal of Clinical & Diagnostic Research, 8*(12), ZE25–ZE29.

Nguyen, L., & Hur, C. (2016). Proton pump inhibitors and dementia incidence. *JAMA Neurology, 73*(8), 1027–1028.

Nieto-Alamilla, G., Márquez-Gómez, R., García-Gálvez, A. M., Morales-Figueroa, G. E., & Arias-Montano, J. A. (2016). The histamine H3 receptor: Structure, pharmacology, and function. *Molecular Pharmacology, 90*(5), 649–673.

NINDS Fact Sheet. (n.d.). Retrieved January 10, 2019, from https://www.ninds.nih.gov/Disorders/Patient-Caregiver-Education/Fact-Sheets/Tremor-Fact-Sheet

Obermann, K. R., Morris, J. C., & Roe, C. M. (2013). Exploration of 100 commonly used drugs and supplements on cognition in older adults. *Alzheimers & Dementia, 9*(6), 724–732.

O'Neal, J., & Remington, T. (2003). Medication-induced esophageal injuries and dysphagia. *Annals of Pharmacotherapy, 37,* 1675–1684.

Perry, L. (2001). Screening swallowing function of patients with acute stroke. Part one: Identification, implementation and initial evaluation of a screening tool for use by nurses. *Journal of Clinical Nursing, 10*(4), 463–473.

Persuad, R., Garas, G., Silva, S., Stamatoglou, C., Chatrath, P., & Patel, K. (2013). An evidence-based review of botulinum toxin (Botox) applications in non–cosmetic head and neck conditions. *Journal of the Royal Society of Medicine Short Reports, 4*(2), 10.

Richelson, E., & Souder, T. (2000). Binding of antipsychotic medications to human receptors: Focus on newer compounds. *Life Sciences, 68*(1), 28–39.

Risacher, S. L., McDonald, B. C., Tallman, E. F., West, J. D., Farlow, M. R., Unverzagt, F. W., & Gao, S. J. (2016). Association between anticholinergic medication use and cognition, brain metabolism, and brain atrophy in cognitively normal older adults. *JAMA Neurology, 73(6),* 721–732.

Roy, N., Stemple, J., Merrill, R., & Thomas, L. (2007). Dysphagia in the elderly: Preliminary evidence of prevalence, risk factors, and socioemotional effects. *Annals of Otology, Rhinology & Laryngology, 116*(11), 858–865.

Rudolph, T. (2017). Antipsychotic (non)selectivity: A setup for swallowing and side-effects in seriously ill elderly adults. *Journal of the American Geriatric Society, 65*(12), 2564–2565.

Ruxton, K., Woodman, R., & Mangoni, A. (2015). Drugs with anticholinergic effects and cognitive impairment, falls and all-cause mortality in older adults: A systematic review and meta-analysis. *British Journal of Clinical Pharmacology, 80*(2), 209–220.

Sacket, D. (1989). Rules of evidence and clinical recommendations on the use of antithrombotic agents. *Chest, 95,* 2S–4S.

Sarris, J., & McIntyre, E. (2017). Herbal anxiolytics with sedative actions. In D. Camfield, E. McIntyre, & J. Sarris (Eds.), *Evidence-based herbal and nutritional treatments for anxiety in psychiatric disorders.* Cham, Switzerland: Springer.

Schiele, J., Quinzler, R., Klimm, H., Pruszydlo, M. G., & Haefeli, W. E. (2013). Difficulties swallowing solid oral dosage forms in a general practice population: Prevalence, causes, and relationship to dosage forms. *European Journal of Clinical Pharmacology, 69*(4), 937–948.

Seeman, P. (2002). Atypical antipsychotics: Mechanism of action. *Canadian Journal of Psychiatry, 4,* 27.

Sera, L., & McPherson, M. (2012). Pharmacokinetics and pharmacodynamics changes associated with aging and implications for medication therapy. *Clinics in Geriatric Medicine, 28*(2), 273–286.

Setacci, C., Sirignano, A., Ricci, G., Spagnolo, A. G., Pugliese, F., & Speziale, F. (2015). A new ethical and medico-legal issue: Vascular surgery and the postoperative cognitive dysfunction. *Journal of Cardiovascular Surgery (Torino), 56*(4), 607–615.

Sirois, P. A., Aaron, L., Montepiedra, G., Pearson, D. A., Kapetanovic, S., Williams, P. L., . . . Oleske, J. M. (2016). Stimulant medications and cognition, behavior, and quality of life in children and youth with HIV. *Pediatric Infectious Disease Journal, 35*(1), 12–18.

Sittironnarit, G., Ames, D., Bush, A. I., Faux, N., Flicker, L., Foster, J., . . . Martins, R. N. (2011). Effects of anticholinergic medications on cognitive function in older Australians: Results from the AIBL study. *Dementia and Geriatric Cognitive Disorders, 31*(3), 173–178.

Sonies, B. (1997). Swallowing disorders and rehabilitation techniques. *Journal of Pediatric Gastroenterology & Nutrition, 25,* 32–33.

Spechler, S., & Castell, D. (2001). Classification of oesophageal motility abnormalities. *Gut, 49*(1), 145–151.

Spieker, M. (2000). Evaluating dysphagia. *American Family Physician, 61*(12), 3639–3648.

Strange, P. (2001). Antipsychotic medications: Importance of dopamine receptors for mechanisms of therapuetic actions and side effects. *Pharmacological Reviews, 53,* 119.

Straumann, A., & Katska, D. (2018). Diagnosis and treatment of eosinophillic esophagitis. *Gastroenterology, 154*(2), 346–359.

Sugawa, C., Takekuma, Y., Lucas, C., & Amamoto, H. (1997). Bleeding esophageal ulcers caused by NSAIDs. *Surgical Endoscopy, 11*(2), 143–146.

Swanson, L. (2014). *Neuroanatomical terminology: A lexicon of classical origins and historical foundations.* New York, NY: Oxford University Press.

Tan, E., Lexomboon, D., Sandborgh-Englund, G., Haasum, Y., & Johnell, K. (2018). Medications that cause dry mouth as an adverse effect in older people: A systematic review and meta-analysis. *Journal of the American Geriatrics Society, 66*(1), 76–84.

Tian, X., Zhou, J., Zeng, Z. Shuai, T., Li-Juan, Y., Li, M, Wang, Y., . . . Song, G. (2015). Cetuximab in patient with esophageal cancer: A systematic review and meta-analysis of randomized controlled trials. *Medical Oncology, 32,* 127.

Tiwari, P., Dwivedi, S., Singh, M. P., Mishra, R., & Changy, A. (2017). Basic and modern concepts on cholinergic receptor: A review. *Asian Pacific Journal of Tropical Disease, 3*(5), 413–420.

Turnheim, K. (1998). Medication dosage in the elderly: Is it rational? *Drugs Aging, 13*(5), 357–379.

Tolosa, E., Martí, M. J., Valldeoriola, F., & Molinuevo, J. L. (1998). History of levodopa and dopamine agonists in Parkinson's disease treatment. *Neurology, 50*(6), S2–S10.

Wilkinson, G. (2005). Drug metabolism and variability among patients in drug response. *New England Journal of Medicine, 352,* 2211–2221.

Williams R. T. (1972). Hepatic metabolism of medications. *Gut, 13*(7), 579–585.

Wright, D., Chapman, N., Foundling, M., Greenwall, R., Griffith, R., Guyon, A., & Merriman, H. (2015). *Guideline on the management of adults with swallowing difficulties.* Leeds, UK: Rosemont Pharmaceuticals. Retrieved from www.rosemontpharma.com/sites/default/files/20150911_adult_dysphagia_full_guideline_clean_approved_sept_15.pdf

Wright, J., Jarman, R., Connolly, J., & Dissmann, P. (2009). Echocardiography in the emergency department. *Emergency Medicine Journal, 26*(2), 82–86.

Yang, S. (2017). Current evidence from post-stroke aphasia. *Brain & NeuroRehabilitation, 10*(2), e15.

Zaninotto, G., Ragona, R., Briani, C., Costantini, M., Rizzetto, C., Portale, G., . . . Parenti, A. R. (2004). The role of botulinum toxin and upper esophageal sphincter myotomy in treating oropharyngeal dysphagia. *Journal of Gastrointestinal Surgery, 8*(8), 997–1006.

Zografos, G., Georgiadon, D., Thomas, D., Kaltsas, G., & Digalakis, M. (2009). Medication-induced esophagitis. *Diseases of the Esophagus, 22*(8), 633–637.

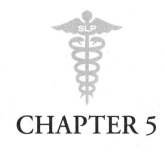

CHAPTER 5

Infection Control Precautions for the Speech-Language Pathologist

Jacqueline Daniels and Kristie A. Spencer

INTRODUCTION

Speech-language pathologists working in all health care settings will treat patients with potentially infectious diseases. Although standard precautions should be used with all patients, additional transmission-based precautions might be added, depending on the type of infectious process encountered. The Centers for Disease Control and Prevention (CDC) recommends usage of precautions combined with immunoprophylaxsis (such as the yearly flu shot and hepatitis B vaccine), as critical steps in preventing spread of disease both to the SLP and between patients receiving services (CDC, 2018). It is important to follow all recommended precautions and to consult with colleagues specializing in infectious diseases when necessary.

STANDARD PRECAUTIONS

Standard precautions were designed to be just that—standard. They are procedures that should be used every time, with every patient. SLPs may unknowingly come in contact with infectious diseases in people who are not yet experiencing outward symptoms, particularly when working in the home and outpatient environments. Application of standard precautions is the best approach to minimize exposure and spread of infection. All SLPs should implement universal precautions, such as thorough hand hygiene, usage of appropriate personal protective equipment, and proper disinfectant or sterilization of shared materials, along with cough etiquette. Cough etiquette incorporates covering a sneeze/cough, performing hand hygiene if warranted, wearing a surgical mask during respiratory illness, and maintaining a greater than three-foot distance from others, if possible, when sick. Although safe injection and lumbar puncture practices are also included in standard precautions, they are less applicable for the SLP's scope of practice. Visitors to the health care setting should also follow standard precautions, including wearing a mask if respiratory infection is suspected.

TRANSMISSION-BASED PRECAUTIONS

When an infectious disease is suspected or known, transmission-based precautions are implemented based on knowledge of how the disease is transmitted. Three categories of precautions include contact, droplet, and airborne, and each has a set of recommendations for patient management. Necessary personal protective equipment is often found in isolation carts stationed outside of the patient's room when in the hospital setting, and should be provided for home health SLPs as well. Masks, such as N95 respirators, require a fit test for the proper size, and should be checked on a yearly basis. When treating patients with viruses that are vaccine-preventable, such as chicken pox, measles, and smallpox, a vaccinated SLP should deliver services if possible. In addition, neutropenic precautions (also known as reverse precautions), may be implemented for immunocompromised patients who do not have an infectious disease, but who are highly susceptible due to their reduced immunity. Use of proper sterilization for reusable equipment, or use of disposable materials, should be considered, particularly for patient's requiring transmission-based precautions. Table 5–1 summarizes the general types of precautions and corresponding personal protective equipment (PPE).

Table 5–2 expands upon elements of Standard Precautions and represents the minimum infection prevention expectations for safe care in outpatient settings. According to the CDC (2016), outpatient care is defined as care provided in facilities where patients do not remain overnight (e.g., hospital-based outpatient clinics, nonhospital based clinics, physician offices, urgent care centers, ambulatory surgical centers, public health clinics, imaging centers, oncology clinics, behavioral health clinics, and physical therapy and rehabilitation centers). Compared to inpatient acute care settings, outpatient settings have historically lacked infrastructure and resources to support infection prevention. Careful adherence to standard precautions on a daily basis is critical to prevent spread of infection and transmission of diseases. Table 5–3 highlights several contagious infection and disease processes with the associated precautions to be implemented by health care providers.

Table 5–1. Summary of Standard and Transmission Based Precautions With Corresponding Personal Protective Equipment

Type of Precaution	Description	Potential Personal Protective Equipment
Standard	Includes Universal Precautions such as hand hygiene, cough etiquette, safe injection practices, and special practices for lumbar punctures	• Gloves, mask, gown, eye protection, and so forth • Safe disposal for soiled linens, dressings and used needles • Proper disinfectant for shared equipment or materials
Transmission-Based Precautions		
Contact	Used for known or suspected infections that can be transmitted via direct contact from one person to another or indirectly from a contaminated surface, including clothing, to person	• All standard precautions • PPE, including gloves and gown, mask with eye protection if splashing is a concern; don PPE upon room entry. • Private room if possible • Limit transport and movement of patients outside of room • Use disposable or dedicated patient-care equipment
Droplet	Type of contact precaution, used when infectious material survives in and is transmitted via respiratory droplets; can be transmitted both through air and on surfaces	• All standard precautions • Put a mask on the patient, especially during transport. • Private room if possible • PPE, including mask, gloves, eye shield, and gown. Don mask upon entry to patient room.
Airborne	Used with microorganisms that can be dispersed through the air over long distances without face-to-face or close contact for transmission	• All standard precautions • Airborne infection isolation room (AIIR) • Fit-tested, NIOSH-approved N95 or higher respirator • Limit transport outside of room to essential services only • Immunize susceptible persons as soon as possible following unprotected contact with vaccine-preventable infections (e.g., measles, varicella)
Neutropenic or Reverse (Thom, Kleinberg, & Roghmann, 2013)	Implemented for patients who have neutropenia (an abnormally low count of a type of white blood cell) as they are immunocompromised generally as a result of chemotherapy	• Standard precautions including mask, even when healthy, avoid sick contacts, including visitors

Source: CDC, 2017a.
Note: PPE = personal protective equipment.

Table 5–2. Summary of Standard Precautions in Outpatient / Ambulatory Care Settings

Preventative Measure	Rationale	Recommendation	Source
Hand Hygiene	Critical to reduce risk of spreading infection	**When:** • Before and after contact with patient • After contact with objects in immediate vicinity • After contact with bodily fluids or contaminated surfaces • Before touching clean site during patient care • After removal of Personal Protective Equipment **What:** • Soap and water if contact with bodily fluids • Soap and water if patient with known/suspected norovirus or *Clostridium difficile* • Otherwise, alcohol-based hand rub	CDC guidelines, Version 2.3 (2016a)
Personal Protective Equipment (PPE)	Wearable equipment intended to protect from exposure to infectious agents, such as gloves, masks, and gowns	**When:** • Facilities should train health-care providers when to use, and how to select, PPE • PPE should be removed and discarded prior to leaving patient care area **What:** • Wear **gloves** for *potential* contact with bodily fluids or contaminated equipment, for example, oral mechanism examination, feeding/swallowing assessment and intervention. • Remove or change gloves and perform hand hygiene when moving between dirty and clean procedures, even on the same client. Wash hands thoroughly after removing gloves. • Wear **gown** to protect skin/clothing if contact with bodily fluids is *anticipated.* Do not wear the same gown for the care of >1 patient. • Wear **mouth, nose and eye protection** if *likely* to encounter sprays of bodily fluid.	CDC guidelines, Version 2.3 (2016a) Interorganizational Group for Speech-Language Pathology (March, 2010)

Preventative Measure	Rationale	Recommendation	Source
Respiratory Hygiene/ Cough Etiquette	Infection prevention at first point of encounter with the facility (e.g., reception and triage areas); targeted primarily at patients and those accompanying the patient. Applies to anyone with signs of illness entering a facility.	At entrance to facilities, must post signs about respiratory infections and provide infection prevention items (masks, alcohol-based hand sanitizer, tissues, etc.). Health care providers should be educated on the importance of infection prevention measures and encourage patients to abide by measures to contain respiratory secretions.	CDC guidelines, Version 2.3 (2016a)
Cleaning and Disinfecting Environmental Surfaces	Policies and procedures needed for routine cleaning and disinfection, especially for surfaces likely to become contaminated with pathogens (e.g., bedrails, doorknobs).	**When:** • Routine. Policy and procedure needed for spills of infectious material **What:** • Cleaning—Scrubbing with a surfactant or detergent / ultrasonic cleaner, and so forth • Disinfecting—Choose EPA-registered disinfectants	CDC guidelines, Version 2.3 (2016a)
Cleaning and Disinfecting Reusable Medical Devices	All reusable medical devices must be cleaned and maintained according to manufacturer's instructions to prevent patient-to-patient transmission of infectious agents.	**Critical items: Come in contact with bloodstream or sterile body tissues. Must be sterile prior to use** • SLP example: flexible and rigid scopes used for stroboscopy or endoscopy, suction tubes **Semi-critical items: Come in contact with mucous membranes or nonintact skin.** High-level disinfection prior to reuse • SLP example: mouthpieces, laryngeal mirrors, ear nozzles/pieces **Noncritical items: May come in contact with intact skin but not bodily fluids.** Low- or intermediate-level disinfection • SLP example: stethoscopes, assessment, and therapy materials, therapy toys, and so forth.	CDC guidelines, Version 2.3 (2016a) Interorganizational Group for Speech-Language Pathology (March, 2010)

Table 5–3. Transmission and Precaution Summary for Commonly Occurring Infections

	Classic Presentation	Transmission	Recommendation Precaution Action	Source
Clostridium difficile (C. diff)	Most commonly affects older adults in hospitals Watery diarrhea, fever, loss of appetite, nausea, abdominal pain/tenderness Risk of disease increases in patients with antibiotic exposure, proton pump inhibitors, GI surgery, long length of stay in health care setting, serious underlying illness, immunocompromising conditions, advanced age	C. diff is shed in feces; any surface, device, or material (commodes, bathtubs, rectal thermometers) that becomes contaminated with feces may have C. diff spores. These spores are transferred to patients mainly via the hands of health care providers who have touched a contaminated surface.	Standard Precautions Contact Precautions	Centers for Disease Control and Prevention (CDC), 2012
Influenza (flu)	Usually comes on suddenly; can experience fever, chills, cough, sore throat, runny/stuffy nose, muscle aches, headache, and fatigue. Some have vomiting/diarrhea (more common in children).	People with flu can spread it to others up to six feet away. Spread mainly by droplets when people with flu cough, sneeze or talk. Less often, a person might get flu by touching a surface that has flu virus on it and then touching their own mouth, nose, eyes.	Standard Precautions Droplet Precautions Health care providers who develop fever and respiratory symptoms should be instructed not to report to work or, if at work, stop patient care activities and don a facemask. Providers should be excluded from work until at least 24 hours after they no longer have a fever without use of fever-reducing medicine. Encourage flu vaccines.	CDC, 2018a

	Classic Presentation	Transmission	Recommendation Precaution Action	Source
Measles	An acute viral, respiratory illness characterized by fever, malaise, cough, inflammation of mucous membranes in the nose, and conjunctivitis, followed by a maculopapular rash. The rash typically appears 14 days after exposure.	Measles is one of the most contagious of all infectious diseases. The virus is transmitted by direct contact with infectious droplets or by airborne spread when an infected person breathes, coughs, or sneezes. Measles virus can remain infectious in the air for up to two hours after an infected person leaves an area. Patients are considered contagious from 4 days before the rash appears to 4 days after.	Standard Precautions Airborne Precautions Infected people should be isolated for four days after developing the rash. Measles can be prevented with a vaccine. Although it is largely considered eliminated in the United States, outbreaks continue to occur each year, mainly from nonvaccinated people or people from outside of the U.S. People exposed to measles who do not have immunity should be offered postexposure prophylaxis (vaccine or immunoglobulin) or be excluded from the setting. This may provide some protection or modify the clinical course of disease among susceptible individuals.	CDC, 2018b
Mumps	Inflammation of parotid glands; can also be asymptomatic, especially in young children	Respiratory droplets and saliva	Five-day isolation period after onset of parotitis for persons with mumps in community or health care settings Standard precautions Droplet precautions Health care providers with no mumps immunity, who are exposed to patients with mumps, should be excluded from duty from the 12th day after exposure through the 26th day after last exposure.	CDC 2007 Guidelines for Isolation Precautions. Mumps update, 2017c

continues

141

Table 5–3. *continued*

	Classic Presentation	Transmission	Recommendation Precaution Action	Source
MRSA (Methicillin-resistant *Staphylococcus aureus*)	A type of staph bacteria that is resistant to many antibiotics. MRSA skin infections often appear as wounds or boils that are red, swollen, painful, or that have pus or other drainage. MRSA can cause bloodstream infections, pneumonia and surgical site infections, and can lead to sepsis and death.	Contact with an infected wound or by sharing personal items that have touched infected skin.	Standard Precautions Contact Precautions	CDC, 2015
Pneumonia (community acquired)	Infection from virus, bacteria, or fungi that inflames the air sacs in one or both lungs; (air sacs often fill with fluid or pus), causing cough with phlegm, fever, chills, difficulty breathing, and fatigue. Most serious for people older than 65 years of age and younger than 2 years of age, as well as people with weakened immune system or other health problems.	Can be spread in a number of ways. Viruses and bacteria can infect the lungs if they are inhaled. They may also spread via airborne droplets from a cough or sneeze. Pneumonia may also spread through the blood, especially during or shortly after birth.	Standard Droplet	Mayo Clinic, 2018 World Health Organization, 2016 Mandell et al., 2007
Shingles (Herpes zoster)	Painful, blistering rash that develops on one side of the face or body; The rash usually clears within 2 to 4 weeks. Can include fever, headache, chills, and upset stomach.	Shingles cannot be passed from one person to another. However, the virus that causes shingles can spread from a person with active shingles to cause chickenpox in someone who have not had chickenpox or who have not received the chickenpox vaccine.	Cover the rash. Avoid contact with people who have not had the vaccine/chickenpox, particularly pregnant women, low birth weight infants, and people with weakened immune systems, until rash has developed crusts.	CDC, 2017b

REFERENCES

Centers for Disease Control. (2016a). *Guide to infection prevention for outpatient settings: Minimum expectations for safe are.* Version 2.3.

Centers for Disease Control. (2016b). *Healthcare-associated infections: Clostridium difficile infection.* Retrieved from https://www.cdc.gov/hai/organisms/cdiff/cdiff_infect.html

Centers for Disease Control and Prevention. (2017a). *Infection control: Transmission-based precautions.* Retrieved from https://www.cdc.gov/infectioncontrol/basics/transmission-based-precautions.html

Centers for Disease Control and Prevention. (2017b). *Shingles (Herpes zoster).* Retrieved from https://www.cdc.gov/shingles/index.html

Centers for Disease Control and Prevention. (2017c). *Mumps update.* Retrieved from https://www.cdc.gov/infectioncontrol/guidelines/isolation/index.html.

Centers for Disease Control and Prevention. (2018a). *Influenza.* Retrieved from https://www.cdc.gov/flu/index.htm

Centers for Disease Control and Prevention. (2018b). *Measles (Rubeola).* Retrieved from https://www.cdc.gov/measles/hcp/index.html

Centers for Disease Control and Prevention, National Center for Immunization and Respiratory Diseases. (2018). Retrieved from https://www.cdc.gov/flu/healthcareworkers.htm; https://www.cdc.gov/hepatitis/HBV/VaccAdults.htm#section1

Interorganizational Group for Speech-Language Pathology and Audiology. (2010, March). *Infection prevention and control guidelines for speech-language pathology.*

Mandell, L. A., Wunderink, R. G., Anzueto, A., Bartlett, J. G., Campbell, J. D., Dean, N. C., . . . Whitney, C. G. (2007). Infectious Diseases Society of America/American Thoracic Society consensus guidelines on the management of community-acquired pneumonia in adults. *Clinical Infectious Diseases, 44,* S27–S72.

Mayo Clinic. (2018). *Pneumonia.* Retrieved from https://www.mayoclinic.org/diseases-conditions/pneumonia/symptoms-causes/syc-20354204

Thom, K. A., Kleinberg, M., & Roghmann, M. C. (2013). Infection prevention in the cancer center. *Healthcare Epidemiology, 57,* 579–585.

World Health Organization. (2016). *Pneumonia.* Retrieved from http://www.who.int/news-room/fact-sheets/detail/pneumonia

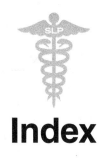

Index

Note: Page numbers in **bold** reference non-text material.